P9-BJJ-787

HEALTH&WEIGHT-LOSS BREAKTHROUGHS 2013

HEALTH&WEIGHT-LOSS BREAKTHROUGHS 2013

FROM THE EDITORS OF **Prevention**®

RODALE

This book is intended as a reference volume only, not as a medical manual.
The information given here is designed to help you make informed decisions about
your health. It is not intended as a substitute for any treatment that may have been
prescribed by your doctor. If you suspect that you have a medical problem,
we urge you to seek competent medical help.

The information in this book is meant to supplement, not replace, proper exercise training.
All forms of exercise pose some inherent risks. The editors and publisher advise readers to take
full responsibility for their safety and know their limits. Before practicing the exercises in this
book, be sure that your equipment is well-maintained, and do not take risks beyond your level of
experience, aptitude, training, and fitness. The exercise and dietary programs in this book are
not intended as a substitute for any exercise routine or dietary regimen that may have been
prescribed by your doctor. As with all exercise and dietary programs, you should get your
doctor's approval before beginning.

Sex and Values at Rodale

We believe that an active and healthy sex life, based on mutual consent and respect between
partners, is an important component of physical and mental well-being. We also respect that sex
is a private matter and that each person has a different opinion of what sexual practices or levels
of discourse are appropriate. Rodale is committed to offering responsible, practical advice about
sexual matters, supported by accredited professionals and legitimate scientific research.
Our goal—for sex and all other topics—is to publish information that empowers people's lives.

Mention of specific companies, organizations, or authorities in this book does
not imply endorsement by the author or publisher, nor does mention of specific companies,
organizations, or authorities imply that they endorse this book, its author, or the publisher.

Internet addresses and telephone numbers given in this book were accurate
at the time it went to press.

© 2013 by Rodale Inc.

All rights reserved. No part of this publication may be reproduced or transmitted in any form or
by any means, electronic or mechanical, including photocopying, recording, or any other
information storage and retrieval system, without the written permission of the publisher.

Prevention is a registered trademark of Rodale Inc.

Printed in the United States of America

Rodale Inc. makes every effort to use acid-free ♾, recycled paper ♻.

Photo credits are on page 352.

Book design by Carol Angstadt

ISBN 978-1-60961-926-8

2 4 6 8 10 9 7 5 3 1   hardcover

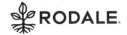

We inspire and enable people to improve their lives and the world around them.
For more of our products, visit **prevention.com** or call 800-848-4735

CONTENTS

PART 3
Fitness Moves

PART 4
Nutrition News

PART 5
Mind Matters

PART 6
Beauty Breakthroughs

INTRODUCTION

ook younger, feel better, live smarter—here's how! We've consulted the top experts, read the medical journals, tested the products, tried out the exercises, and tasted the recipes to make sure that this book is filled with simple solutions to help you. With the advice tucked between the two covers of *Health & Weight-Loss Breakthroughs 2013*, you can take simple steps to look, feel, and live your best!

This book is filled with the latest health breakthroughs on weight loss, nutrition, fitness, mind matters, and beauty. Here, you'll find smart strategies to apply these medical breakthroughs to your own life.

In Part 1: Health Breakthroughs, you'll discover the top latest amazing innovations—and how they can enhance your health and well-being. From heart disease to cancer to head injuries—we've got you covered. You'll also learn about critical screening tests and the latest breakthroughs in alternative medicine.

In Part 2: Weight-Loss Wisdom, you'll discover the latest information about losing weight. Learn how eating the right types of calories can help you lose weight. Take our challenge to be fit and fabulous in just 4 weeks. And best of all, find out why the best diet might actually be no diet at all.

Turn to our Bonus Weight-Loss Cookbook for this year's best *Prevention* recipes. They're delicious, nutritious, and easy to make. Our favorites are the Baked German Apple Pancake with Cherry Preserves, Roasted Vegetable Soup,

Dreamy Creamy Macaroni and Cheese, Grilled Rib-Eye Steak with Mustard Sauce, and Chocolate Cherry Cupcakes with Vanilla Bean Frosting.

You'll get movin' and groovin' with Part 3: Fitness Moves. Lace up the right way with our simple shoe solutions. Pack a workout into your overfull day by getting twice the workout in half the time. And use our simple target toning to blast off your pesky problem spots.

Then in Part 4: Nutrition News, you'll learn how to eat better than ever. We focus on two of our favorites: the incredible, edible egg and the all-American burger. You'll also read about the new way to go vegetarian. Get inspired by mothers against junk dining. And don't miss our special report on genetically modified foods.

Feeling down? Anxious? Exhausted? Check out the new strategies and innovations in Part 5: Mind Matters. Get inspired on your journey in pursuit of happiness. Find out how you can go from hectic to happy. And solve your own personal energy crisis.

You'll look great after following the tips in Part 6: Beauty Breakthroughs. First take our Defy-Your-Age Challenge. Then make yourself beautiful from head to toe: Make every day a great hair day. Give your skin a youthful, beautiful glow. Pamper your feet with our pedi-cure.

We've filled *Health & Weight-Loss Breakthroughs 2013* with the latest and greatest health and weight-loss news and information. We wish you great health and happiness!

Part 1

HEALTH
BREAKTHROUGHS

CHAPTER 1

The Bionic Heart

Heart disease kills more Americans than any other illness. But a new game-changing medical breakthrough can now keep women active and vital—and will one day make heart transplants virtually obsolete.

Joyce Thomas of Rockville, Maryland, enjoys a full, active life. She holds down a demanding job as a bookkeeper for a condo complex, goes dancing with her husband, and likes eating out with friends.

Nothing unusual here, except that Thomas has no pulse.

No, she's not the heroine of the latest sci-fi flick or vampire TV series. She's an average 53-year-old woman whose heart, just a year and a half ago, was operating at only a quarter of its normal capacity.

Enter a cutting-edge new medical intervention, a left ventricular assist device (LVAD). Most people have never heard of an LVAD—unless they happened to be paying close attention a few years ago when former vice president Dick Cheney, a survivor of five heart attacks, had one installed. Scientists have been working on the technology (basically a scaled-down version of a jet engine) for several decades, but it wasn't until the mid-1990s that there was a model that could be implanted inside a patient's chest cavity, and it wasn't until 2005 that the device was tailored to be small enough to fit the average woman.

The LVAD was originally intended as a stopgap measure to keep patients alive while they waited for a heart transplant to become available. The 2-year survival rate for people with end-stage heart failure had been 8 percent; after the LVAD first became available, the rate jumped to 23 percent. And although the new, petite model, the HeartMate II, has been FDA-approved for only a few years, it's already been okayed as a "destination therapy," meaning it can be used in patients who aren't good transplant candidates. The real hope is that one day LVADs may replace heart transplants altogether. In the meantime, they're saving women's lives.

WHAT MAKES A HEART PUMP TICK

A healthy human heart pumps about 2,000 gallons of blood through the body daily, delivering oxygen and nutrients to organs and tissues. But if damaged or weakened by heart disease or a heart attack, it can't pump with the force required to get the organs what they need. That's what's meant by the term *heart failure*, which affects more than 5 million Americans (approximately 2.6 million of them women), with about half a million more diagnosed every year. It results in shortness of breath, fatigue, chest congestion, swelling of the legs, and kidney problems. Ultimately, heart failure can be fatal.

That's where the LVAD comes in. The pump is about the size of a D battery, with two flexible tubes, one of which attaches to the aorta, the other to the left ventricle. Once implanted, the pump takes over the function of the left ventricle—the largest and hardest-working chamber of the heart—pushing blood out through the aorta to the rest of the body. The device is powered by special batteries that are connected to a controller, which attaches to a power cord that extends from the LVAD through a permanent incision in the patient's abdomen.

Unlike the heart you were born with, however, the LVAD motor moves blood continuously, not with a pumping rhythm. That's why most patients, like Joyce Thomas, have no pulse. As a result, they have to wear medical alert tags at all

A DAY IN THE LIFE OF AN LVAD PATIENT

Living with an LVAD is not for the faint of heart: It takes constant commitment from the patient and a support team of friends and family.

The pump's power cord exits the patient's body through an open incision, which must be kept clean, dry, and bandaged at all times to prevent infection. Because Joyce Thomas's husband, Paul, wasn't able to take time off from work to attend the extensive training sessions, her sister, Debby, who lives nearby, cleans the incision and changes the dressing twice a week. The process takes about 45 minutes.

What's more, water is kryptonite to the apparatus, so swimming and strolling in the rain are out. Thomas has a waterproof bag to protect her batteries in the shower, but she finds it too cumbersome, so instead, she fills the tub, sits on the edge, and gives herself a thorough sponge bath. But the most nerve-racking reality is the 12-hour-max life span of her LVAD batteries—without which Thomas would die within minutes. The power cord coming out of her abdomen connects to a controller that attaches to the battery packs, which she carries in a fanny pack or shoulder bag. The importance of carrying a spare set of batteries at all times is drilled into LVAD patients: Their lives depend on it.

During the day, just carrying around the 6-pound battery pack (plus the spare) is a substantial burden—so Thomas gets help. "If Paul and I are going out, he carries the pack for me," Thomas says. "When I'm at work, and we go to lunch, my friends may offer to help. But I enjoy being independent."

At night, Thomas has to sleep with her power cord connected to a main unit in her bedroom that plugs into a regular wall socket. "If I want to go to the kitchen, I have to put the batteries back in," she says, but a 20-foot-long cord allows her enough mobility to get as far as the bathroom without batteries. "And in terms of being intimate, it hasn't affected us at all," she adds.

Despite the challenges, all that cooperation has heartwarming bonuses: Thomas says her marriage is stronger than ever. "It's brought us closer together."

times—so if they're knocked unconscious in an accident, for example, emergency workers won't assume that they're dead.

In her early twenties, Thomas became unexpectedly ill, and doctors discovered damage to her cardiac muscle and told her she had congestive heart failure. A normal heart pumps out between 55 and 70 percent of its blood with each beat; heart failure may be diagnosed when that "ejection fraction," as it's called, drops below 45 percent, and Thomas's was at about 20 percent. Once she'd recovered, she managed to keep her condition relatively stable under the care of various cardiologists, who put her on meds, including the beta-blocker carvedilol and digoxin, to regulate her heart function. For years, these proved effective in strengthening her heart muscle.

Thomas also diligently ate a healthy diet and exercised regularly.

All seemed well until she reached age 40, when her condition deteriorated, and her heart function again dropped. Even getting a pacemaker to control her irregular heartbeat didn't halt the progress of the disease. Then, finally, her condition became critical. She felt exhausted and weak, coughed constantly due to fluid in her lungs, and had trouble sleeping.

"She was making gurgling noises at night," recalls her husband, Paul, a manager for CVS. She couldn't even climb the three steps to enter her house without help.

His resources exhausted, Thomas's cardiologist recommended that she try Washington Hospital Center, one of the country's top cardio-care facilities, located in nearby Washington, DC. Before she'd even made an appointment, Thomas woke up one August morning to find she could barely breathe.

"I asked my husband to drive me to the hospital, but I was terrified the doctors would say, 'Joyce, there's nothing more we can do for you,'" she recalls.

As scared as they were, the couple passed the closest hospitals and drove 45 minutes to Washington Hospital Center. It's lucky they did. The doctors there determined that Thomas was in dire shape, but not eligible for an immediate heart transplant. However, this cardiac center offered another option, one that only two hospitals in the area provided: The facility's specially trained surgeons could attach a 3-inch LVAD to Thomas's heart to pump her blood for her. Thomas was so ill that the operation—though less strenuous than a transplant—wouldn't be easy, nor would the substantial lifestyle changes she and her family and friends would have to make. But it gave her a second chance. And she'd be alive.

Thomas was in such critical condition that the doctors told her she had to decide right away, before her heart deteriorated further. Her ejection fraction was down to a mere 15 percent; there was no question. Two days later, on a Thursday, she had the LVAD implantation surgery. The following Monday, she was already sitting up in the intensive care unit.

"I quickly started to feel so good," she says. The first time she went for a walk outside her hospital room, she remembers, "My doctors were standing out in the hallway, and they all started clapping."

WHAT HAPPENS WHEN YOUR HEART WON'T EVER STOP?

LVAD technology is still so new that no one's caught up yet with the ethical and legal questions it presents. If a heart pump patient has a stroke or other condition that causes multiple organ failure or brain damage, the LVAD keeps on working, meaning that—legally speaking—the patient doesn't die. Should the pump be disconnected? And if so, when—and who makes the decision?

Ideally, the answer is the patient herself.

"It's crucial to begin to discuss some of these contingencies with the patient before they happen," says Lynne Warner Stevenson, MD, professor of cardiovascular medicine at Harvard Medical School and director of the cardiomyopathy and heart failure program at Brigham and Women's Hospital in Boston. A recent Mayo Clinic study of 14 patients whose heart pumps were disconnected when the patients were in dire condition found that even when they had left end-of-life instructions, none of them mentioned their LVADs. In 12 of these cases, the families and medical staff had to make the harrowing choice to disconnect the LVAD. The other two patients were still able to ask to be allowed to die.

The study's authors concluded that "carrying out such requests is permissible" because death results from the underlying heart disease. The idea is that the LVAD should be treated like any other life-extending apparatus, such as a breathing tube. But that might offer scant comfort for families faced with such a painful choice. To spare them guilt and uncertainty, Dr. Stevenson asks her patients to make end-of-life decisions before the LVAD is implanted.

In November, 3 months after the life-saving surgery, Thomas was back at home and at work—and healthier than ever.

"I feel great, better than I have in years," she says. "I'm full of energy, and I can work around the house and go for walks with my husband again."

Even though only 15,000 people so far have received an LVAD—and only approximately 7,000 have the new, smaller HeartMate II—the heart pump is undoubtedly a game changer.

"We're talking about a tremendous improvement in survival rates," says Samer Najjar, MD, medical director of heart failure, heart transplantation, and mechanical circulatory support programs at Washington Hospital Center. Earlier this year, a study showed an 85 percent 1-year survival rate for LVAD patients awaiting transplant, which rivals the 88 percent 1-year rate for those receiving transplants—until now, the gold standard for heart failure treatments.

SIMPLER CPR

You can stop a heart attack before it has the chance to damage the heart: There's been a dramatic change to the recommended CPR guidelines. If you see someone suddenly collapse from apparent cardiac arrest, call 911, and give hard and fast chest compressions until emergency help arrives, according to new guidelines from the American Heart Association.

"Because the mouth-to-mouth step can be intimidating, bystanders often panic and do nothing," says Michael Sayre, MD, associate professor of emergency medicine at Ohio State University in Columbus and an author of the guidelines. "But giving chest compressions can double or triple a victim's odds of survival."

This technique works without training, and it's also more effective. It quickly distributes oxygen already in a victim's bloodstream. Giving breaths first (the classic CPR method still recommended for a near-drowning or choking victim and for children) can mean a harmful delay for heart attack victims. For a tutorial, visit handsonlycpr.org.

"LVADs have already reduced the need for heart transplantation, and I have no doubt that a total artificial heart will eventually be perfected," says Steven E. Nissen, MD, chairman of the department of cardiovascular medicine at the Cleveland Clinic.

The LVAD's original manufacturer, Thoratec, estimates that between 50,000 and 100,000 heart failure patients a year could benefit from the device. But only about 135 of the 5,000-some hospitals in this country have invested in the extensive training, equipment, and personnel necessary to implant heart pumps—whether for patients awaiting heart transplants or as destination therapy—and provide the follow-up care needed.

Because LVAD procedures are concentrated in such a small handful of hospitals, many doctors—even cardiac specialists—are unaware that this treatment option exists.

"The task for us is really to educate cardiologists," Dr. Najjar says. "So many more patients could benefit from this technology than now do."

Thomas is living proof of what a difference the device can make. Accepting the challenges that come with an LVAD is easy because she simply feels so much healthier. Smiling as she pats the battery pack she must keep with her at all times, she says, "As for carrying this thing around? It's just like a purse. Except it's keeping me alive."

CHAPTER 2

Special Alert: A Head Injury You Should Never Ignore

A hit on the head can be far more dangerous for grown women than for men or children. Read—and save—this special report.

One May morning 3 years ago, Julie Supple was walking her golden retriever in her New Jersey neighborhood when he lunged at another dog. Supple, then 46, slipped on the grass and fell with a thud, banging her head on the ground. Right away, she felt nauseated and had a pounding headache, but she brushed herself off and headed home. She had to get her daughter to school and herself to work.

Thankfully, that meant the hospital, where Supple, a nurse practitioner for a neurosurgery practice, had morning rounds.

"I still felt sick and headachy but was trying to act normal. I didn't want to believe that anything was seriously wrong."

Her colleagues insisted she get a CT scan of her head, which would detect any bleeding. Though it came back normal, they admitted her to the hospital because she was vomiting, having crushing head pain, and was too wobbly on her feet to walk straight. The diagnosis: severe concussion, a brain injury that's not detected through imaging tests but, rather, by assessing the degree of symptoms. It would take 4 months for Supple to recover and return to work.

YOUR CONCUSSION CARE KIT

A bump on the head could be a bigger deal than you think. Here are some rules to follow.

Call Your Doctor

If you have any of these symptoms:

- Headache
- Dizziness
- Trouble concentrating
- Feeling overstimulated by lights and noises
- Memory loss, especially of the accident itself

Your doctor might want to perform neurological tests of your strength, balance, reflexes, and memory to rule out other brain damage—or might send you to the hospital for further testing.

Call an Ambulance

If you experience any of the following:

- Temporary loss of consciousness
- Vomiting
- Severe headache
- Trouble speaking or seeing clearly

"I didn't realize at the time how sick I was," she says now.

Supple is one of the lucky ones, says her boss, John Knightly, MD, co-medical director of the Atlantic Neuroscience Institute Concussion Center at Overlook Hospital in Summit, New Jersey. She began to rest and recover right away, perhaps avoiding a worse outcome.

"But many women ignore their concussion symptoms, thinking things will get better," he says. "That's a real health gamble."

- Numbness in your limbs
- Symptoms that persist or worsen

At the emergency department, a CT scan might be performed to assess you for brain bleeds. Be vigilant about noting any changes in mood, behavior, or cognitive abilities for a month after you hurt your head. Mark your calendar so you don't forget.

Give Yourself Time to Rest and Recover

The only cure for a concussion is physical and mental rest. "If you hurt your knee, you wouldn't run," says John Knightly, MD, co-medical director of the Atlantic Neuroscience Institute Concussion Center at Overlook Hospital in Summit, New Jersey. "You have to treat your brain the same way."

Don't take aspirin or ibuprofen, which increase your risk of brain bleeds. For pain relief, take acetaminophen or ice your head.

Don't push yourself mentally. Don't do anything that gives you a headache or makes you tired. Stay home from work if your doctor recommends it.

Don't exercise. A subsequent blow to the head—second impact syndrome—can cause severe brain swelling and affect blood flow to the brain, which can be fatal.

More than 90 percent of concussion symptoms improve within 3 to 4 weeks, but more serious cases can take longer. To avoid delayed healing or secondary injuries, wait for your doctor's all-clear before returning to your normal activities.

TROUBLE AHEAD

Bumping your noggin can be serious business: The risk of stroke is 10 times greater for 3 months following a concussion or other traumatic brain injury, according to new research published by the American Heart Association. The danger: Injury-caused clots may loosen over time, leading to a stroke, says study author Herng-Ching Lin, PhD.

WOMEN AT RISK

Some 1.2 million people get concussions every year, most of them mild. Another 500,000 suffer more dangerous problems, including severe concussions like Supple's, as well as brain bleeds such as contusions and hematomas, the latter of which killed actress Natasha Richardson in 2009. But even a minor concussion—when the brain shakes around in the skull—is far from harmless. If it doesn't heal, it could lead to memory loss or chronic sensitivity to bright lights and noise, says Dr. Knightly, or even increase your risk of dementia decades later.

Although recent media attention has focused on concussions in pro football players, research indicates that adult women may be especially at risk.

"Women have smaller frames and neck muscles than men, which may make them more prone," says Daniel Labovitz, MD, assistant professor of neurology at the Albert Einstein College of Medicine in Bronx, New York. Once a woman is injured, the effects can be much more dire. In a 2010 study, women took longer than men to recover from concussions; this was especially true among women of child-bearing age.

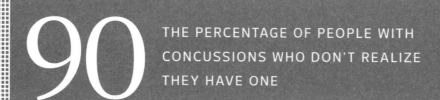

90 THE PERCENTAGE OF PEOPLE WITH CONCUSSIONS WHO DON'T REALIZE THEY HAVE ONE

35

THE PERCENTAGE OF HEAD INJURIES CAUSED BY SLIPS AND FALLS, THE LARGEST SINGLE CAUSE

Fluctuating hormones might affect how the brain recovers from trauma, says Jeffrey Kutcher, MD, a sports neurologist at the University of Michigan in Ann Arbor. Other research found that female soccer players performed worse on neurological testing after concussions than men with comparable injuries.

What's more, women and men alike (especially those who take blood thinners) are more prone to brain bleeds from head injuries than children are. Brain matter shrinks over time—and when there's less brain in your skull, there's more room for it to bounce upon impact, creating a greater risk of bleeding.

That's why it's so important to take any head injury seriously—and to continue to monitor symptoms for days, weeks, and even months afterward. Some, like a headache or confusion, might seem minor, but if they worsen over time, they can signify bleeding, which usually requires surgery.

"Don't assume you just feel 'off,'" says Anthony Alessi, MD, a neurologist in Norwich, Connecticut. "When in doubt, seek medical attention."

For news about kids and concussions, go to prevention.com/concussion.

CHAPTER 3

Four Screening Tests Not to Fear

Health screenings can save lives, yet many women are afraid of the pain. Discover ways to make them less scary and more comfortable.

Millions of Americans delay—or even skip—key health screenings such as mammograms, MRIs, and colonoscopies for just one simple reason: fear. Because overcoming your dread of these exams can literally save your life, we gathered experts' best tips for getting through them with minimal discomfort—plus news about the latest high-tech alternatives.

MAMMOGRAM

What it does: By taking x-rays of a flattened breast, mammography can detect 80 to 90 percent of breast cancers—even ones too tiny to be detected by a manual breast exam. A Swedish study found that regular mammograms can cut the death rate of women in their forties by up to 29 percent.

The fear factor: Starting from near your underarm, a technician will tug your flesh until it's positioned between two plastic paddles and then compress it, which can hurt, especially if your breasts are small, dense, or sensitive. Most mammograms take only about 10 seconds of compression per view—just 40 seconds total.

Ace That Test!

Apply a topical painkiller. In one study, women who applied an over-the-counter 4 percent lidocaine gel to their breasts before their mammograms reported significantly less pain during the test. Two hours before your appointment, apply no more than 1 ounce of gel; within 1 hour, wash thoroughly with warm water. (Gel ingredients can interfere with image results.)

Are there any alternatives? For women at average risk of breast cancer,

---

EASE THE STRESS OF ANY TEST

Stress doesn't have to make having a procedure even worse. De-stress with these natural approaches.

TRY ACUPUNCTURE. This ancient technique tamps down stress hormones while boosting feel-good endorphins, says Lixing Lao, PhD, professor of family and community medicine in the Center for Integrative Medicine at the University of Maryland School of Medicine in Baltimore. "Several acupuncture points on the body work on general anxiety," including the ear, shoulder, and stomach, says Dr. Lao, who advises scheduling an appointment a few days before your exam. Your insurance might cover acupuncture; if not, a 1-hour session will cost $60 to $120, on average.

CALM YOUR MUSCLES. Begin progressive relaxation exercises in the waiting room, advises Jeanne van Gemert, a mind/body therapist at Duke Integrative Medicine in Durham, North Carolina. Tense your shoulders for 5 seconds, then release; do your back next; repeat several times. "When you're stressed, you unconsciously tighten your muscles," she explains. "Clenching fully and then relaxing fully can be a big relief."

mammograms are the standard, says Elizabeth Thompson, president of Susan G. Komen for the Cure, headquartered in Dallas. For women with very dense breasts or a family history of breast cancer, ultrasound, a painless procedure that uses sound waves to detect abnormalities, is sometimes used along with mammograms. Insurance rarely covers it as a solo preliminary screening.

COLONOSCOPY

What it does: This procedure is the most effective way for your doctor to look for polyps and other precancerous growths in your colon. If she finds any, she can usually remove them painlessly on the spot through the scope itself. The procedure can last from 30 minutes to an hour.

The fear factor: It's not the thought of having a long, flexible tube with a tiny camera on the end (a scope) inserted in one's rectum that makes most people cringe. (You'll be sedated.) It's the colon-clearing prep you have to do the day before. After being on a 24-hour clear liquid diet, you must drink either one-half or a full gallon of a salty prep liquid at least 7 hours before the exam. The drink will make you empty your bowels repeatedly until there's nothing but clear liquid coming out. This can sometimes cause abdominal pain, nausea, and vomiting.

Ace That Test!

Get a head start. The less you have in your gut before you start flushing out your colon, the easier the process will be.

"I approach the prep as if it were a cleansing diet," says Dede Cummings, coauthor of *Living with Crohn's & Colitis.* "A few days beforehand, I start eating smaller, lighter meals, like skinless baked chicken, rice cakes, and applesauce."

Drink the liquid in 1 day. If you can, schedule your appointment for the afternoon, and then begin drinking your prep liquid that morning. Although the American College of Gastroenterology suggests drinking half the prep at night and half the next morning, a recent study at Thomas Jefferson University shows that patients who saved the entire prep for the morning of the procedure experienced less abdominal pain and had uninterrupted sleep because they weren't running to the bathroom all night.

Keep a chaser on hand. Wash down the drink with water, Gatorade, or ginger ale, advises Sunanda Kane, MD, professor of medicine and staff gastroenterologist at the Mayo Clinic in Rochester, Minnesota.

"You can't dilute the prep with another drink in the same cup, but you can drink them side by side," she says. Your colon must be completely clear to get an accurate reading, so follow prep guidelines exactly, says Harminder Singh, MD, assistant professor of gastroenterology at the University of Manitoba Winni-

COULD YOU BE OVER-XPOSED?

Despite the hubbub over radiation emitted by newer airport scanners, medical imaging tests like x-rays account for **36** percent of our exposure to manmade radiation. Because radiation has been linked to cancer risk, the US Nuclear Regulatory Commission caps it at 50 millisieverts (mSv) a year for people working with radioactive material, which is a level you can reach with just a few tests. (An airport scanner delivers 0.00003 to 0.0001 mSv per scan.) If your doctor orders an imaging test, ask why, and if there are alternatives. Here is the radiation emitted by common tests.

RADIATION SOURCE	DOSE PER SCAN (MSV)
Full set of dental x-rays	0.005
Chest x-ray	0.1
Mammogram	0.36
Abdominal x-ray	0.7
CT scan of the head	2
Cardiac calcium scoring	2
Upper GI x-ray	6
Barium enema	8
CT scan of the abdomen/pelvis	10
Virtual colonoscopy	10
Whole-body CT scan	10
Heart angiography	20

peg. This is especially key for women: Dr. Singh and fellow researchers concluded that women are 31 percent more likely to have their cancers missed than men, in part because cancerous lesions in women usually occur in the upper colon, where it's harder for the camera to reach.

Ask for prep pills. If you just can't tolerate the taste of the liquid, the prep is available as a pill. Think of this as a last resort though.

"You have to take 32 tablets in 1 ½ hours," says Carol Burke, MD, director of the Center for Colon Polyp and Cancer Prevention at the Cleveland Clinic, and the sodium phosphates in the pills have been associated with rare but potential kidney damage. But because the risk of kidney damage is smaller than the lifetime risk of colon cancer, in very few cases (less than 1 percent), Dr. Burke offers the pills to prep-resistant patients, with informed consent.

Are there any alternatives? In a virtual colonoscopy, an MRI or CAT scan takes several cross-sectional x-rays of your colon. It's fast and noninvasive—though you still have to do the full prep. But while some private insurance companies cover this alternative, it's not covered by Medicare unless there's a medical reason the patient can't undergo traditional colonoscopy (if there's excessive twisting or scarring of the colon, for example, or the patient can't tolerate anesthesia). Also, if the doctor spots a polyp, you'll need a regular colonoscopy to remove it anyway, says Dr. Burke.

Upon FDA approval, which could happen as soon as late 2013, those at low risk (no family history of colon cancer or personal history of polyps) may have a new screening option. The Cologuard test is an at-home kit that allows a patient to collect a small amount of stool and mail it to a lab for analysis. The test will look for DNA changes associated with precancerous and cancerous polyps. You'll need a traditional colonoscopy only if the test shows DNA change.

ENDOSCOPY

What it does: Upper endoscopy is similar to colonoscopy, except that the scope is inserted down your esophagus while you're sedated to examine your esophagus, stomach, and beginning of your small intestine. Endoscopy is used to investigate the cause of specific symptoms, such as chronic reflux, swallowing difficulty, and upper abdominal pain. Just as with colonoscopy, your doctor can also remove any polyps on the spot.

"It's important to look at patients over age 60 who have reflux or sudden pain swallowing, because the older esophagus is less sensitive—so by the time you feel pain, any disease that is present may be more severe," says Lawrence Brandt, MD, emeritus chief of gastroenterology at Montefiore Medical Center in Bronx, New York.

A diagnostic endoscopy should take about 5 to 7 minutes; if you have any polyps, it might take a few minutes longer.

The fear factor: There's little preparation; you just have to fast for 6 to 8 hours before the test.

"Many patients are concerned that they'll gag or throw up when the scope is inserted," even though they'll be sedated, says Dr. Brandt. Those reactions rarely happen, but because the doctor inserts air while the scope is down, you might feel pressure. This usually goes away within a few hours; afterward, you might also have a slight sore throat.

Ace That Test!

Schedule it for first thing in the morning. You naturally fast while you're sleeping, so Dr. Brandt suggests eating dinner as usual the night before and scheduling an early-morning procedure.

Ask for an anesthetic spray. If you can't shake the fear of gagging, request an anesthetic spray before the procedure for peace of mind.

Treat your throat gently afterward. If your throat feels sore from the scope, Dr. Brandt recommends eating soft foods for the rest of the day. Ease back in with yogurt, gelatin, and ice pops, and skip anything irritating, like spicy or hard foods.

Are there any alternatives? An old-fashioned upper GI series—in which you ingest a chalky barium drink and your esophagus, stomach, and first part of your small intestine are x-rayed—is still an option, but there's also a newer development: With a capsule endoscopy, you swallow a large pill-size capsule that has a miniature camera inside. As the camera moves painlessly through your entire GI tract, it transmits images to a receiver you wear in a vest—no sedatives

THE GYN MISTAKE SMART WOMEN MAKE

If you've checked "gynecologist visits" off your to-do list because you're finished having kids, you could be making a fatal mistake. Late-stage cervical cancer is most often found in women over 50, according to a new report from the Centers for Disease Control and Prevention. This is a reality directly attributable to the fact that women this age don't always get regular Pap tests, which can detect the cancer early. To protect yourself, have an annual checkup and a Pap every 3 years if you've had three normal results in a row.

required. You can go home or to work while the camera travels through your system; it is eventually eliminated in your stool, and you can flush it away.

The drawback? Because it allows only for diagnosis (not treatment) and has potential complications, capsule endoscopy is used and covered by insurance only when traditional colonoscopy and endoscopy have failed to locate the source of pain or bleeding.

MRI

What it does: MRI (magnetic resonance imaging) uses a strong magnetic field and radio waves to create cross-sectional images of your body. Because it shows organs, soft tissue, and bones, doctors use MRI to help diagnose everything from torn ligaments to brain tumors and cancer. You'll be sent headfirst into an enclosed tube and must lie still while listening to the taps and thumps of the scanner. (You'll be offered earplugs.) It can take from 10 minutes to over an hour.

The fear factor: An MRI doesn't cause any physical pain, but the psychological challenge of lying still in a narrow tube might make a person feel very claustrophobic.

Ace That Test!

Listen to a favorite book. "Go to another place in your mind," says Jeanne van Gemert, a mind/body therapist at Duke Integrative Medicine in Durham,

North Carolina. You can't take your iPod (or anything metal) into the MRI, but most centers have sound systems, so you can bring a CD of your favorite novel for them to play. Closing your eyes and visiting India or Italy can make the time go faster. Even a CD of your favorite music can keep you relaxed.

Imagine you're going home. Numerous studies link guided imagery to lower anxiety during medical treatments, including surgery, chemotherapy, and MRI.

"I often advise patients to imagine the trip home from the hospital," says Donald Wood, a certified registered nurse anesthetist in Florida. "Picture every street you drive down and all the landmarks along the way, like the church on the corner. It can be a great distraction." Or fantasize about a vacation, family reunion, shopping spree—whatever makes you happy.

Take anti-anxiety medication. If mental distractions won't ease your claustrophobia, ask your doctor to prescribe an anti-anxiety drug before the MRI.

GOOD HEALTH IS IN THE BAG

Certainly, life comes with its share of bumps and bruises—both big and small. Prep your trusty tote with these essentials from emergency physicians Melissa Barton, MD, and Lee Benjamin, MD.

SUPERGLUE: No kidding! It can help heal a shallow cut. Align the skin edges together, rub a thin layer of glue over them, and hold for 30 seconds.

A TEA BAG: For split lips, press a damp black tea bag to the area. Its tannins help halt bleeding in mouth and gum tissue.

ALCOHOL-BASED HAND SANITIZER: Dole some out when you're in a germy situation and need clean hands, such as before eating at a mall food court.

UNCOATED ASPIRIN: It's not just for headaches. If you have heart attack symptoms, it could be lifesaving. Chew one and seek emergency care.

NASAL SPRAY: To stop a nosebleed quickly, use a nasal spray containing oxymetazoline (such as Afrin), and then apply pressure for 10 minutes.

TWEEZERS: They can remove splinters, bug stingers, and glass from cuts.

BANDAGES: If you get a blister while on the run, your feet will thank you.

Are there any alternatives? At some "open MRI" centers, you can stand, sit, or even watch TV while you get scanned. But these tubeless machines aren't always ideal, says Jeffrey Weinreb, MD, professor of radiology at the Yale University School of Medicine. "Open MRIs generally use low magnetic fields, which do not yield the same quality of images as the high magnetic fields in closed scanners," he explains. Low magnetic images may be adequate during a routine scan of the brain (for chronic headaches) or knee, Dr. Weinreb says, but for other exams, such as those looking to detect cancerous tumors, a high magnetic scan is recommended. The good news: Closed scanners are now being built with shorter, wider tubes and require only your head to be enclosed if you have a brain scan.

CHAPTER 4

The Big O

Here's everything you didn't think you needed
to know about ovarian cancer.

What if there were a cancer that had virtually no symptoms (or so everyone told you)? What if there were no routine screenings (or ones your insurer would cover)? What if any symptoms you tried to report were dismissed by your doctor as vague or benign complaints? And what if, when that cancer was finally detected, it would almost certainly be too late to save you, and you'd be told you had only about 5 years to live? Now, what if that cancer could have been found, could have been treated, and could have been cured with very little muss and fuss? Would you be mad as hell? Sure you would—and you should be. There's no "what if" about it. This is the reality of ovarian cancer today.

Each year, about 21,880 American women of all ages and races are diagnosed. And while every cancer exacts a devastating toll, ovarian cancer is disproportionately deadly. One out of five women with breast cancer ultimately dies from it (looking at the combined rate for all stages of the disease), and survival has improved dramatically over the years. But ovarian cancer takes the lives of two out of every three women diagnosed—and that hasn't changed for 3 decades.

It doesn't have to be this way. If ovarian cancer is caught early, in Stage I, when it's still confined to the ovary, a woman has up to a 94 percent chance of long-term survival. But today, more than 70 percent of women still aren't diagnosed until the disease has advanced to Stage III or IV, meaning that only 18 to 45 percent of them will live another 5 years. The reason? We aren't effectively screening for ovarian cancer, and even after symptoms appear, women—and too often their doctors—frequently don't recognize them. So we're told to take antacids or wait it out—giving the cancer time to spread. All this has to change, starting now. With you.

WHERE WE ARE NOW

When Nancy Baez of Allendale, New Jersey, developed mild indigestion in June 2007, the then 47-year-old chalked it up to the Cuban food she'd eaten on vacation. Two months later, while she was visiting the Outer Banks, North Carolina, her stomach trouble flared up, and she took over-the-counter antacids. But by September, she not only had indigestion, she was exhausted too.

"I remember thinking, I'm getting old," she says. Her primary care doctor took her vitals, ordered an external abdominal ultrasound to check her gallbladder (which was fine), prescribed stronger pills for her gastric symptoms, and told her to call in 2 weeks if she didn't feel better. One week later, Baez phoned her doctor and said, "I'm having trouble breathing." The next day, a CT scan revealed she had Stage IIIC ovarian cancer, and her tumors were so big that they were pressing against her lungs. "I was in complete shock," recalls Baez.

Stories like this—of tumors not detected until the prognosis is grave—are still the norm with ovarian cancer, which is the deadliest of the reproductive cancers. The only routine check most of us ever get for it is our annual pelvic exam. While a pelvic is great at unearthing many problems, from cervical cancer to infections, ovarian cancer is decidedly not one of them. More often than not, a gynecologist performing the exam is unable to feel your ovaries at all, let alone find any cancer in them. That's due to simple anatomy. Soft and walnut-shaped, the ovaries are suspended on either side of the uterus, deep within your core, and they're no more than 1½ inches in diameter. What's more, after a woman reaches menopause—when her risk of ovarian cancer rises—her ovaries begin to shrink and get even harder to feel. Researchers in one study could manually feel the ovaries in only 30 percent of women over 55.

Making things worse, the symptoms of ovarian cancer—such as indigestion, bloating, pelvic pain, and an urgent need to urinate—are such common indicators of less dangerous conditions that, until recently, doctors didn't realize that the disease had symptoms, calling it the "silent killer." That, at least, has changed—because finally a researcher asked women themselves what they had experienced.

In January 2007, Barbara Goff, MD, director of gynecologic oncology at the University of Washington in Seattle, astounded the medical world by finding that the silent killer wasn't really so silent after all. In a groundbreaking study, Dr. Goff and her team reported that the 149 women they followed shared a startlingly similar constellation of symptoms in the months leading up to their ovarian cancer diagnoses. While these warning signals do mimic less serious conditions, such as heartburn or indigestion, Dr. Goff also figured out what set them apart from such comparatively minor problems: Rather than just having occasional rounds of bloating or stomach pain, the women who had ovarian cancer experienced their symptoms 12 or more times a month during a period of 12 months or less.

The medical establishment quickly embraced Dr. Goff's work, and as a result, today when a woman goes to her doctor with a complaint listed on this "symptom index," and ovarian cancer is suspected, insurers generally cover the follow-up diagnostic tests. The index has had a major impact on getting women treated more quickly after symptoms appear.

But while the index is a significant breakthrough, it's not a screening test.

In the absence of screening, it's important that women know the symptoms of ovarian cancer so they can see the doctor in a timely fashion, says Cynthia A. Gelb, director of the Centers for Disease Control and Prevention's Inside Knowledge campaign (cdc.gov/cancer/knowledge), an initiative to educate women about gynecological cancers. If they signal ovarian cancer, any of these symptoms would likely occur as often as three times a week over a period of several months to a year.

- Pain in your pelvis or abdomen
- A strong or frequent need to urinate
- Abdominal bloating
- Difficulty eating or a tendency to feel full quickly

If you have any of these symptoms in the time frame given above—or you have a family history of reproductive cancer—and suspect ovarian cancer, tell your doctor and ask for an exam, a transvaginal ultrasound, and/or a blood test.

By the time a woman is experiencing symptoms, the cancer could already be advanced. What we need now is an early detection test that women can have routinely to discover cancer at its very earliest stages, before symptoms even appear.

HOPE ON THE HORIZON

Nobody's saying that finding a good screening test is easy. Like any other early detection tool, one for ovarian cancer has to meet some tough criteria. According to standard medical practice, such a test has to be sensitive—meaning it has to be able to identify the cancer early, so there's a low likelihood of false positives. It has to be specific—it must find any existing cancer, minimizing false negatives. It has to be affordable, so that women can take it often enough to catch these fast-growing tumors. It has to be safe. And above all, it has to have incontrovertible clinical evidence that it saves lives—enough lives to be worth the time and money it will require from women, doctors, and insurers: Otherwise doctors won't recommend it, and insurers won't cover it.

It's a tall order. But we've managed to develop screening tests for other cancers, and it's paid off: The Pap test slashed the death rate from cervical cancer by nearly 70 percent. And dedicated researchers do have real leads on screening tests that could have a similar impact on ovarian cancer, some of which are already in clinical trials. Here are some of the leading candidates right now.

Transvaginal Ultrasound (TVU)

This simple, painless procedure has a lot going for it, because it's so easy to perform. Here's how it works: Your doctor inserts a probe into your vagina to get a detailed image of your ovaries. If there's a mass, TVU (also called transvaginal sonography, or TVS) will find it. That's why it's already used as a diagnostic tool to help rule out or confirm ovarian cancer in women who have symptoms or significant risk factors. But right now, it's not used as a standard screening test for all women in the way that mammograms are, despite the fact that no other reliable method of finding an ovarian tumor early exists. And unless it is

HOW YOU CAN JOIN THE FIGHT

Support the search for an early detection tool and a cure for this deadly disease during September, National Ovarian Cancer Awareness month— and the rest of the year too. Here's how.

Contact your congressional representative and stress your concern about ovarian cancer research dollars being cut.

Wear teal, the official color of ovarian cancer awareness, on September 2— Teal Day—to show your support.

Donate to ovarian cancer research groups, including the National Ovarian Cancer Coalition (ovarian.org), the Ovarian Cancer Research Fund (ocrf.org), and the Ovarian Cancer National Alliance (ovariancancer.org).

For more ways to help, log on to prevention.com/ovarian.

approved for routine use by all women, insurance companies won't pay for it, and many doctors won't suggest it for screening purposes.

John R. van Nagell Jr., MD, director of gynecologic oncology at the University of Kentucky Markey Cancer Center in Lexington, is hoping to provide the proof that routine sonograms for all women will save lives through the university's Ovarian Cancer Screening Research Program. Since 1987, he and his team have used TVU on more than 37,000 women.

"So far, we've found about 500 [masses], and about 60 were cancer," he says. "We're looking for needles in haystacks, but we are finding them."

One case in point: Suzi Shoemaker of Midway, Kentucky. In April 2006, Shoemaker, then 50, was the healthy, happy owner and manager of a horse farm. She'd recently had her annual pelvic and believed all was well. Although she didn't think she was at risk, she signed up to participate in Dr. van Nagell's project, and the TVU detected a "large structure" on her left ovary. Within 24 hours, a surgeon had operated on Shoemaker, found that the mass was malignant, and removed a golf ball–size tumor. The cancer was at Stage I; Shoemaker's prognosis was good; and 5 years later, she's still cancer free. But had she not had the TVU, the tumor most likely would not have been detected until it reached Stage III or IV, and she might well not have lived to see her 55th birthday.

One complaint lobbed by critics about TVU is that sometimes when a mass is found via ultrasound, a doctor can't determine whether it's cancerous with-

A CANCER WARNING NOT TO IGNORE

Nonmelanoma skin cancer is the most common and curable cancer, but it could also be a canary in the coal mine, report researchers at the Medical University of South Carolina: People who get this cancer may be nearly 50 percent more likely to develop other cancers later in life. And if you're diagnosed between ages 25 and 44, you might face an even greater rise in risk, possibly because the early onset indicates a genetic predisposition to cancer. If you've had this disease, be vigilant about getting other cancer screening tests.

out performing surgery to biopsy it, and operating is always a risk. However, given how lethal ovarian cancer is, many women might decide that a biopsy is well worth it even if it finds only a harmless cyst.

"I wouldn't have minded the surgery even if my tumor had been benign," says Shoemaker. "I would just have been tremendously relieved and grateful."

Still, to combat such false positives, at the National Ovarian Cancer Early Detection Program in New York City, researchers are studying whether pairing TVU with a contrast agent can improve the specificity of the findings. During a preliminary study, women had TVU and, if a suspicious mass was found, were then injected in the arm with the contrast agent, which reached the ovaries within 30 seconds and gave the technician a 3-minute mini film of the blood flow in and out of the possible tumor.

"The flow for a malignant mass is much slower than it is for a benign one," explains David Fishman, MD, director of the program and professor of obstetrics, gynecology, and reproductive science at Mount Sinai Medical Center in New York City.

TVU is also inexpensive, costing about $100 if you pay out of pocket, but another argument against it is that the price is too high when you consider how many women must undergo TVU in order for just one cancer to be discovered. Dr. van Nagell disagrees, pointing out that the cost of medical treatment for a patient with Stage III ovarian cancer is somewhere between $200,000 and $300,000. Besides, he adds, "what we're talking about is the value of a woman's life."

A Better Blood Test

A blood test called CA-125 is already being used to see if women with ovarian cancer are responding to chemotherapy or if their cancers have come back. Researchers are exploring whether the test—which measures certain protein (biomarker) levels that become elevated when ovarian cancer is present—could be used for routine screening. But CA-125 can rise in women for many reasons other than ovarian cancer, including benign tumors, endometriosis, fibroids, pelvic inflammatory disease, hepatitis, and breast cancer. And CA-125, like He-4 (another biomarker being studied), doesn't always spike if a woman has Stage I or II ovarian cancer. Some researchers are investigating whether

A PRESIDENT'S PROMISE

President Barack Obama lost his mother to ovarian cancer in 1995, when she was just 52. Here's what he told *Prevention* magazine in an exclusive statement:

"Experiences like my mother's are far too common. Ovarian cancer still claims more lives than any other reproductive cancer. That's why my administration is committed to developing effective screening, improving treatments, and defeating this disease.

"While we continue to promote awareness of ovarian cancer and advance its diagnosis and treatment, it falls to all of us to look out for the women we love. I encourage all women, especially those over age 55 or with a family history, to protect your health by understanding risk factors and discussing possible symptoms with your health care provider. And talk to your loved ones: Encourage them to gather the facts and protect their health."

combining the two biomarker tests might give a more accurate result. If they're successful, the end product may be affordable too: Each test currently costs somewhere between $29 and $138.

TVU Plus CA-125

Researchers at MD Anderson Cancer Center in Houston recently showed that a careful combination of a yearly blood test with a TVU chaser if the biomarker levels rise could hold promise. For 8 years, Karen Lu, MD, professor of gynecologic oncology, studied 3,238 women age 50 and older, using an approach called the Risk of Ovarian Cancer Algorithm (ROCA), which has established normal, intermediate, and high-risk CA-125 levels. A woman with normal levels continues to receive an annual CA-125 test. If her biomarker climbs into the intermediate risk range, she gets a follow-up CA-125 test 3 months later; if it's in the high-risk range, she's given a TVU.

Dr. Lu's study is a smaller version of a major United Kingdom project that may answer the question, once and for all, of whether ROCA can save women's lives. Called the UK Collaborative Trial of Ovarian Cancer Screening, the study is massive—researchers are following 202,638 postmenopausal women. If the results, due to be reported in 2014, show that ROCA is reliably accurate, this might be the answer we need.

CASH FOR CURES

"Recent research has been so promising that I hope in 5 to 10 years, we'll see a screening tool that will pick up ovarian cancer at an earlier stage, when cure rates are substantially better," says Dr. Lu. "An early detection test seems more within reach now than it did when I started my career 20 years ago."

So what's it going to take to push all this promising research on screening tests over the hump so we can start saving lives? In a word, money. And soon there may be even less of that available.

Funding for research on ovarian cancer comes from a patchwork quilt of federal agencies (which gave nearly $132 million, or 92 percent) and nonprofit organizations (nearly $12 million, or 8 percent). One of the biggest contributors of federal money has, for years, been the Department of Defense. It gave $20 million to ovarian cancer research in fiscal year 2011, a $1.25 million increase over 2010. However, that's still just a fraction of what the DOD contributes toward research on other cancers, such as breast and prostate.

Even more worrisome, however, some members of Congress now want to group all federal cancer research funding under the National Cancer Institute (NCI). If that happens, women's advocates fear ovarian cancer research might get lost in the shuffle, given that the disease affects fewer people than does breast, prostate, colorectal, or lung cancer. But the size of the population suffering from a disease should not be the measure of how much funding the research gets, according to Thomas Herzog, MD, director of the division of gynecologic oncology at Columbia University Medical Center in New York City.

"Considering the incredible mortality and devastation of ovarian cancer, we don't currently fund the research on this disease commensurate with the damage it causes," he says.

Representative Rosa DeLauro (D-CT) is a 25-year survivor of ovarian cancer. Because her tumor was diagnosed only by chance when it was still at Stage I, she understands how urgent the need is for an early detection tool.

"I know firsthand the lifesaving power of basic medical research," she says. "It's one of the reasons I ran for Congress—to help ensure that we maintain the investments in science and technology that saved my own life. But those investments are in very real danger." In addition to the uncertain status of DOD funding right now, according to DeLauro, the current majority in the House of Representatives is slashing basic medical research from its budget, and, she adds, "that means potentially lifesaving medical studies could be put on hold or even stopped completely."

Representatives Ralph Hall (R-TX) and Howard Berman (D-CA) reintroduced in the House the Ovarian Cancer Biomarker Research Act, but it was not enacted. If the bill had become law, the director of the NCI would have been required to help establish and fund Ovarian Cancer Biomarker centers of excellence, which would work on finding an early detection test, as well as on establishing more definitive risk factors.

"Now more than ever, it's critically important that ovarian cancer advocates come together to support this important research," says Sabrina Valvo, director of communications for the Ovarian Cancer Research Fund in New York City. "We have at our disposal such a huge amount of knowledge and technology that was unimaginable just 20 years ago. We are so optimistic that the fight against ovarian cancer can make significant gains in the next few years—if we can just keep the research dollars coming."

MAKE YOUR PC AN MD

A new (free!) service at skinofmine.com lets you upload a photo of a mole, then analyzes its size, color, and borders and rates the likelihood that it could be skin cancer. If your spot looks iffy, the site can put you in touch with a doctor for an online consultation. This costs about $50, depending on where you live.

HANG UP ON CANCER

These days, cell phones seem like a necessity for safety. After all, the time of seeing a pay phone on every corner and in every store is long gone. But ironically, your cell phone might also pose a tremendous health hazard.

Collectively, Americans spend more than 6 billion minutes a day glued to their cell phones. But new science suggests a link between heavy cell phone use (30 minutes or more a day) and an increased risk of a type of brain cancer. And now a brand-new study from the National Institutes of Health reports that the electromagnetic radiation that's given off by a cell phone antenna triggers an increase of brain glucose in the area of the head that's closest to where the cell phone is held.

The health effect of all of this cell phone use, if any, remains unknown. But if you want to minimize your exposure until all the evidence is in, follow these proven safety tips from Devra Lee Davis, PhD, an epidemiologist and author of the book *Disconnect: The Truth about Cell Phone Radiation.*

Try to avoid direct contact with your cell phone during calls. Use the speaker-phone setting or wired hands-free device. Although wireless Bluetooth devices do reduce radiation, they don't eliminate it.

Follow the bars. Radiation exposure increases when a cell phone's signal is weak or when you're traveling in a fast-moving car or train. That's because the phone needs to constantly reconnect to new towers. Wait till you have three or more bars showing before you make your call.

Tell your kids to text. Because their skulls are thinner than adults', children absorb radiation at a higher rate when they hold a phone to their ear. But remind your teens not to text while driving, since that carries even more dangerous risks!

Save the long chats for a noncordless landline or an Internet phone system, like Skype. And when you're on the go, let your fingers do the talking and send a text instead.

CHAPTER 5

Love in the Time of Viagra

Nearly one-fifth of boomer men are taking Viagra, throwing off the sexual tempo in long-term marriages and shuffling the status quo for the newly divorced and dating.

Things that at first seem so simple, so often aren't. "Take a pill, feel better" suddenly becomes complicated. The little blue pill enables older men to sexually respond like 18-year-olds. While men of a certain age are undoubtedly thrilled to have their sexual potency restored, maybe their wives' enthusiasm is a bit more subdued.

What at first glance seems an obvious win-win situation for both husbands and wives can have a raft of unintended consequences. Don't get us wrong: Viagra is a wonder drug. Since the early '90s, when researchers testing a new heart medication called sildenafil discovered that it had a startling side effect in men, erectile dysfunction drugs have become more than a billion-dollar industry. One study conducted by Express Scripts, a pharmacy benefit management company, found that nearly 20 percent of all American men over age 45 have tried them. And since, according to the National Institutes of Health, approximately 5 percent of 40-year-old men and from 15 to 25 percent of 65-year-old men experience ED (for reasons ranging from narrowing of the blood vessels with age to high blood pressure, diabetes, obesity, and neurological problems), these drugs have been a godsend to millions. ED drugs can also, indirectly, be lifesavers. Thirty-four to 70 percent of all men who take antidepressants experience sexual dysfunction as a side effect, and of those who have this problem, almost 90 percent stop taking the antidepressants so their sex lives can go back to normal.

But ED drugs are so readily available, so much a jokey part of the cultural landscape, that few of us really know how they work and what the potential dangers are. This leads to misuse—not so much life-threatening as knuckleheaded.

Essentially, ED drugs work like this: What gives a man an erection is blood flow to the penis. The vessels dilate, and blood flows in. There is an enzyme that counteracts the dilation. ED drugs inhibit that enzyme, allowing dilation to occur more easily and last longer. They can also diminish a man's refractory time, meaning that after orgasm, he can more quickly get an erection again.

The one thing most people know about Viagra and its cohorts is that they are not supposed to be used by men who take nitroglycerin, a common medication for heart patients that also dilates the blood vessels. But ask around. That little piece of knowledge has translated into "Viagra is bad if you have a heart condition."

Not so, says Arthur S. Agatston, MD, a cardiologist and associate professor of medicine at the University of Miami Miller School of Medicine and *Prevention* editorial advisory board member. In fact, Dr. Agatston says, because Viagra keeps the blood vessels from becoming "sticky" and helps blood flow through them smoothly, not just in the penis but throughout the body, in the future, many of us—women included—may end up taking some small amount of Viagra daily, the way we take low-dose aspirin, which has the same nonsticking effect on blood itself.

So when a man takes Viagra, he has to avoid anything that dilates the blood vessels, not just nitroglycerides. Drinking, lying in the sun—both are problematic. Viagra won't give him a heart attack, but, taken with too much alcohol, it could make him pass out, Dr. Agatston says.

UNINTENDED CONSEQUENCES

Perhaps more damaging than ignorance of the physical ramifications of ED drugs is ignorance of their potential interpersonal blowback. When not discussed frankly, Viagra can cause a lot of misunderstanding and hurt between couples.

"There is something about a hard erection that is extremely important to a man's identity," says Steven Lamm, MD, an internist in New York City and author of *The Hardness Factor*. "And of course, most couples would prefer that the man be able to have one. But there are some who may have adjusted to life without sex. Perhaps the woman doesn't really want it anymore, for one reason or another. And for those couples, the introduction of an ED drug can throw them seriously out of sync."

That leads to what is perhaps the biggest complicating factor: the reality that a woman's postmenopause genital health can put her physically at odds with her partner's newfound, drug-assisted prowess. As women age, their hormonal balances change. Reduced estrogen levels often mean less sexual desire but also decreased vaginal elasticity and lubrication, and thus more potential for sex to be painful.

The problem can be especially daunting for older women who are widowed or divorced or just beginning to date after years of being alone or with one man. Certainly this was the case for Marjorie P., a 60-something woman who complained about the drugs on a 50+ Web site: "Men have been saved from their middle-age sexual issues by Viagra and Cialis. They can be 30 again, while I have to deal with the sexual issues of being my age. It's put the world on 'tilt.'" Andrea D., a twice-divorced physician from Santa Monica, California, and an over-50 dater, put it more bluntly. "Viagra has been liberating for men, but unless a woman is taking hormone therapy, she may have vaginal dryness and

(continued on page 44)

GREAT SEXPECTATIONS

A revealing new study has pinpointed the true sources of sexual pleasure for women. Let the findings reignite your sex life—if you dare.

Women haven't been waiting for a lab report to learn that sexual sensation centered on the vagina is different from sensation centered on the clitoris—or on the breasts, for that matter. But apparently this is breaking news to sex researchers, who have only recently confirmed these facts using high-tech brain scans. And if this information comes as a surprise to your partner too, you'll be able to change your sex life in the most satisfying ways imaginable.

This new research comes from Rutgers University, where Barry R. Komisaruk, PhD, has been studying women's sexual response for 3 decades. He and his colleagues have now shown that not only does stimulation of the clitoris, vagina, cervix, and nipples activate distinct brain regions of the genital sensory zone of the cortex but also that titillating one area affects other sexual brain sectors as well.

These findings are especially important to long-standing couples, who all too easily fall into sexual ruts, according to Nan Wise, a certified sex therapist and PhD candidate in Dr. Komisaruk's lab. The same old, same old sex routines don't work for women because female sexuality is nuanced and complex—more like a symphony than a cymbal clang. If your partner's approach to sex is one-note—exclusively focused on your vagina, for example—he's shortchanging your pleasure potential.

"Not every woman likes every type of touch, but there is likely a cumulative effect," says Wise. "For most women, layering three or four types of stimulation could lead to a better sexual experience than enjoying one thing only." The result is that couples now have myriad reasons to try new positions, modes of touch, and means of sexual expression. Release your habits and inhibitions, and let the fun begin.

SHOW AND TELL. In order to defuse some of the tension that can creep into couple conversations about less-than-satisfying sex, consider drawing your partner a personalized pleasure map instead. Laura Berman, PhD, host of *In the*

Bedroom with Dr. Laura Berman, provides her clients with a black-and-white outline of a figure's front and back on a sheet of paper. Circle the areas of the body where you'd like your partner to lavish attention. Also key: Assign each zone a number, which tells your partner what part of your body you want stimulated first, second, third, and so on.

IT'S ALL IN THE WRIST. Some women shy away from breast attention because their husbands don't know how to touch them in a way that feels good. Now that we see how tied in to the brain's sexual pleasure circuit the nipples are, it's time for men to brush up on their technique. "Men tend to touch their partners the way they want to be touched: fast and hard," says Dr. Berman.

"You need to ask him to start slow, caressing the breast gently." The foreplay map will point him in the right direction, but you'll need to refine his efforts by explaining exactly what you want, according to Dr. Berman.

LESSONS IN SELF-LOVE. It helps to try some exploratory masturbation so you know what to ask your partner to do differently in bed. If you've been touching yourself the exact same way since you were a teenager, the time has come to try a new routine. Pick an area you don't usually pay attention to and experiment. When you discover a new sensation you love, show your partner how you like it.

PLAY A HEAD GAME. In long-term relationships, women tend to be tougher to turn on than men, at least in terms of what the sexperts call spontaneous sexual desire. That's the powerful impulse that drives men to come on to their wives regardless of the situation. Many long-married women don't get lusty on the spur of the moment, according to Wise. They need a subtle matrix of mental and physical cues to really get in the mood.

But there are ways to get things cooking. "Women can kick-start sexual desire in themselves if they just start engaging physically," says Wise. That means being open to intimacy even if your mind is in a thousand places and none of them is between the sheets. Your brain will catch up with your body, especially if your hot zones are getting expert attention from a partner specially trained to turn you on.

really not be that interested in the kind of driving, pounding intercourse he's now capable of."

There is also fallout from the erroneous belief that Viagra causes not just greater blood flow but also greater desire. The hormone testosterone is the driving force behind libido; a man with little or no testosterone will not have any desire to have sex, Viagra or no. Moreover, even with normal amounts of testosterone, "Viagra does not just instantly give a man an erection," says Abraham Morgentaler, MD, associate clinical professor of urology at Harvard Medical School and author of *The Viagra Myth*.

"You have to be in a sexual situation—you need to have desire and intent—in order for the drug to work." Dr. Morgentaler tells the story of a patient who was very upset because Viagra didn't do the trick for him. "He said, 'Doc, I followed your directions exactly. I took the pill an hour in advance. Then I watched a baseball game on TV and waited.' The man's wife was in the other room, waiting too; neither of them realized that the drug would be effective only if they were together, doing what couples do."

The misunderstandings cut all ways: Some women think ED drugs make men amorous and that their presence isn't required. "What a lot of women need to be turned on is the feeling that they're desired," adds Virginia A. Sadock, MD, director of the program in human sexuality at New York University Langone Medical Center in New York City. "So with Viagra, they think, 'Oh, it's not me he wants; it's the Viagra talking.' In my practice, I spend a lot of time reassuring them that this isn't the case, and I tell men they must reassure the women too."

Another big issue for many women: ED drugs drastically shorten the interval between climaxing and achieving another erection. Men look at this differently than women do. For them, it's not a bug, it's a feature. And for the woman?

"We want maybe 20 or 30 great minutes of sex," says Susan K., a mother of two in Connecticut. "We don't want an interminable 2 hours." Not to mention the fact that prolonged intercourse, particularly without sufficient lubrication, can do damage. It can lead to vaginal abrasions and even tearing and can expose a woman to the risk of getting yeast infections and—particularly for a woman who is dating or divorced—to sexually transmitted diseases.

There are, too, single women who worry that men with new-and-improved

WHAT ABOUT THE G-SPOT?

The G-spot, the much-debated area on the front wall of the vagina, is the focus of as many rumors as Bigfoot or Elvis. It's supposedly the source of some of the most intense orgasms, and even ejaculation, when manipulated correctly.

"Unfortunately, there's more known about certain areas of outer space than there is about certain areas inside a woman's vagina," says Nan Wise, a Rutgers University researcher and a certified sex therapist in New Brunswick, New Jersey. The existence of the G-spot remains a controversial subject, even though Italian researchers reported pinpointing its location using ultrasound in a small 2008 study. To date, scientific consensus hasn't been reached. But there's no reason not to do some research of your own—no one can blame a girl for trying.

sexual abilities will be less likely to commit to marriage, and wives who worry that their husbands will be more apt to look outside the marriage for sex.

"A partner's Viagra use is now another reason some women give when I ask why they've come to see me," says Miami plastic surgeon Lee Gibstein, MD, who has performed breast implants, face-lifts, and even vaginal rejuvenation on women concerned about turning back the clock.

Which is not to say that Viagra hasn't ever led to straying—but not for the reasons women think. "I've seen problems when a wife or partner objects to ED drugs on the grounds that sex should be natural and spontaneous," says Dr. Morgentaler. So if the man is unable to have erections on his own, and the woman shoots down the idea of a pill, then the guy is really stuck. The relationship can get into trouble, because one person wants sex and the other doesn't or only wants it on her terms.

HELP AND HOPE

So how can you make sure, if ED drugs come into your marriage, that they help rather than hamper your relationship?

"Couples really need to talk about what each partner in the relationship expects," says New York couples counselor Jane Greer, PhD, author of *What About Me?: Stop Selfishness from Ruining Your Relationship*. "The drug can highlight problems about which member of the couple puts him or herself first, which one is thoughtful and which isn't—creating all sorts of conflict."

Adds Andrea, whose own Viagra dating experiences and the experiences of similarly aged friends have ranged from excellent to "emergency care needed": "You have to be crystal clear about what works for you and what doesn't. Because even with someone you really, really adore . . . sometimes you just want to get back to reading your book!"

Moreover, women need to stop lying about what they like and don't like to protect the male ego, because that's a recipe for sexual dissatisfaction.

"Women can cheat themselves out of good sex because they don't take responsibility for their own feelings, both physically and emotionally," says Dr. Sadock. This means: If you need to buy lubricant to make sex more comfortable, do it; if you need to tell him you're perfectly happy having intercourse for a few minutes, do that too.

BRINGING SEXY BACK

It's a touchy subject: Both men and women in long-term relationships report that they want to be having more sex—but aren't. It's important that you find out what's holding you back—and how to close the desire gap.

If you could take a pill daily that would lower your blood pressure, reduce stress, boost your immune system, and promote bonding with your mate, wouldn't you do it? You don't actually need a pill to tap these much-needed benefits. There's another way that's more fun, with no side effects: having sex with your mate. So why do so many couples let their relationships fall into a sex-free zone?

It starts with your pressure-cooker job, on top of your load of household chores. Add your husband's own stressed-out work life, his ailing mother, and some unexpected bills that are throwing off your budget. Pepper the mix with two small (or large) children, and what you have is a recipe for a couple who

THE POWER OF SEXY SURPRISES

You don't have to do gymnastics in bed to bring new thrills to your relationship. Even small breaks in your sex routine—a slightly new position, a different room in your house—can energize your love life, according to Erika Pluhar, PhD, a certified sex therapist in Atlanta. Why? "Eroticism thrives on newness, mystery, and risk," says Dr. Pluhar. So get frisky while improving your health: Sex bolsters immunity and burns calories too.

would just as soon collapse on the couch as shimmy under the sheets.

This scenario is so common that therapists have an acronym for it—DINS, as in "dual income, no sex." And it's not only men who are unhappy about it. According to an Australian study published recently in the *Journal of Sex & Marital Therapy*, fully 28 percent of women ages 35 to 54 who are married or in long-term relationships would like more sex, please. With 53 percent of the men also reporting dissatisfaction, that means at least half of couples are experiencing a "desire gap."

There's an opportunity here. Frequency of sex is intrinsically tied to happiness in a relationship. The National Opinion Research Center at the University of Chicago has consistently found that married couples between the ages of 30 and 59 who describe themselves as "very happy" have sex about 60 percent more often than those who describe their relationship as "not too happy." (That's 78 times a year versus 48.) "But does more sex lead to greater happiness or greater happiness to more sex?" asks Tom Smith, PhD, a senior fellow at the National Opinion Research Center.

Evidence suggests that it works both ways. So to boost your health—and happiness!—here are some tips to help you get your groove back.

Take a shortcut. After a tiring day, anything that helps ignite your sexual energy should become part of your arsenal. For men and some women, soft porn or magazines often do the trick. (So don't feel inadequate if your husband resorts to porn—and don't be embarrassed to use it yourself.) But for many

HOW TO WIN AT THE WHEEL OF HORMONES

It's probably not a surprise how dramatically your hormones affect your life, including your sex life. New research reveals how hormone fluctuations affect your health all month long. Here's how, and why, and how you can make this roller coaster work for you.

Days 1 to 13

YOUR CHOLESTEROL SPIKES. Total cholesterol levels rise by almost 20 percent during the follicular phase, according to a recent study. Book doctor visits at the same time of the month for consistent comparisons.

YOU'RE MORE INJURY-PRONE. New research suggests that hormones might decrease muscle control during this time, making women more susceptible to knee injuries. Jumping exercises can cut your risk.

Days 14 to 15

MULTITASKING IS HARDER. Higher levels of estrogen during ovulation might affect your ability to concentrate. Take extra time to find your keys.

YOU FEEL SEXY! Women are often in the mood when they're most fertile, says Rebecca Booth, MD, an ob-gyn in Louisville.

Days 16 to 28

SYMPTOMS INTENSIFY. If you have an ongoing health issue—such as depression, migraines, or asthma—you might feel worse right before your period, says Dr. Booth.

GUMS ARE SENSITIVE. Surges in progesterone before menstruation can increase gum inflammation and discomfort. Make dental appointments at the start of your cycle, or take a pain reliever first.

CRAVINGS PEAK. Plummeting estrogen causes a dip in your brain's "feel-good" chemicals, making you crave sugar and starch, says Dr. Booth. So treat yourself to a little dark chocolate. You deserve it!

women, romance novels are equally likely to promote passion, says family therapist Michele Weiner-Davis, author of *The Sex-Starved Marriage*. By providing vicarious thrills, they can help generate natural lubrication too. So on your way home from work, pick up a copy of *Voluptuous Vixen* or *Seduce Me at Sunrise*. When you get to the "good bits," you just might be inspired to snuggle up to your husband and try it out with him. By providing vicarious thrills, racy romance novels can help generate natural lubrication.

Be adventurous. It's not only the time crunch but also boredom with the routine that kills passion for most long-term couples—because really, if you were excited about sex, you would make the time, says therapist Esther Perel, author of *Mating in Captivity: Unlocking Erotic Intelligence*.

Variety adds that proverbial spice. But the pursuit of novelty doesn't mean you have to twist yourself into every position in the *Kama Sutra*. The goal of sex is to bond and have fun, not to end up in traction. Try anything that makes you feel naughty or seductive. That might mean role playing ("Professor, I need some extracurricular tutoring") or dressing up like Rhett and Scarlett (forget the hoop skirt and go straight to the corset).

Think like a Realtor. Location, location, location: A change of venue accomplishes two goals. It adds novelty, and it gets you away from the household drudgery and chores that tend to make your husband blend into the domestic scenery rather than appearing to be an enticing sexual being. But don't limit your thinking to a romantic B&B. You'll feel more risqué, says Perel, if you rendezvous at a hotel for a quickie at noon. Spring for a hotel room and reinvent the idea of "room service."

Clear the air. Smoldering resentments, not alleged time pressures, are often the true cause of a diminished sex life. Couples blame each other for placing too much emphasis on children or careers at the expense of the relationship—or for being lazy bums who can't find a job and won't help out around the house. Such attitudes are not exactly turn-ons. Who'd want to cuddle up with someone who's not only not romantic but actually simmering with anger? Rather than relying on a grope in the dark, try opening up lines of communication and making him feel appreciated—and hope the gesture will be reciprocated.

"When people feel understood, they often feel a greater sense of love or passion," says Kenneth Paul Rosenberg, MD, clinical associate professor of psychiatry at Weill Cornell Medical Center in New York City. If you can't solve all your problems, at least come to enough of a truce to give each other pleasure. Problem solving may get easier after that.

Just do it. According to therapists, there are four stages of sex—desire, arousal, orgasm, and return to normal. "But for a lot of people, stages one and two—desire and arousal—can happen in reverse order," says Weiner-Davis. Allow your partner to touch you sexually, whether you're in the mood or not. Nerves that are wired to parts of the brain involved in sexual excitement will be stimulated, and physical arousal will likely follow.

Exercise à deux. Enjoyable activities can help couples bond—and if sharing a hike or a tennis game makes you feel great, you will tend to associate those feelings of exhilaration with your partner. Even going to the gym together on a regular basis can make you feel stronger as a couple. But a more direct turn-on might be yoga. Many studios offer workshops for couples in which you interact with your partner—starting with simply sitting cross-legged on the floor and gazing into each other's eyes.

"Yoga poses bring you into a place of vulnerability and openness, where you're not talking around a problem or blaming each other," explains Becky Jeffers, a yoga therapist and wellness coordinator at North Shore Urogynecology in Park City, Illinois. Other poses involve leaning on each other—feeling your partner's skin, spine, and weight against you—or even sitting in your husband's lap, facing him, with your legs wrapped around him. "Lots of long-term couples try this on their date night or Valentine's Day," she says. "It generates a lot of heat, both physical and sexual." It's a kind of foreplay—and you finish at the same time!

Try a good squeeze. There are other forms of sexual behavior besides intercourse, says Stacy Tessler Lindau, MD, director of the program in integrative sexual medicine for women with cancer at the University of Chicago. She's found that many couples who can't have intercourse for medical reasons tend to spend more time touching, holding hands, and hugging as an alternative way of bonding. But these acts of affection are important for healthy couples too. In a recent study of long-term partners who were together an average of 25 years, the Kinsey Institute for Research in Sex, Gender, and Reproduction at Indiana University found that, yes, sex was important. But frequent kissing and caressing were also predictive of happiness in the relationship—even more for men than for women, says Kinsey director Julia Heiman, PhD. The study didn't examine why, but psychologists note that a loving touch makes you feel desired.

Whatever you do, don't give up. Jenna (not her real name), a 56-year-old salesperson in California, thought her sex life was over when she reached menopause. "I told my husband I was done," she says. "My hormones had crashed. I thought I was never going to have an orgasm again." He took her declaration as a challenge to bring it back—and he did, with a flourish, relying more on manual stimulation than he had before. Now Jenna is brimming with enthusiasm about her reinvigorated sex life. "No one is more surprised than I am," she reports—or more happy to be proven wrong.

CHAPTER 6

The Healing Edge

Complementary and alternative medical treatments are gaining respect and influence in established corridors of health care. Try these healing treatments today.

There's a health care revolution going on, and chances are you're part of it. Across the country, more and more doctors are embracing complementary and alternative medicine, prescribing therapies such as acupuncture and yoga, and dispensing advice on the right way to breathe and eat. Thirty-eight percent of Americans already use integrative practices. And now, countless researchers are proving their benefits.

As a result, there's new hope that patients with various chronic conditions can find relief without surgery or drugs. We salute the most remarkable achievements and individuals who have helped change the way we all take care of our bodies and minds.

Here we discuss some of the most common—and some of the most researched—alternative treatments: acupressure, yoga, massage, meditation, and acupuncture. Could these alternative medical treatments be good for whatever ails you?

ACUPRESSURE
Soothe away stress.

In an exciting new discovery, acupressure (which relies on finger pressure rather than needles) can reduce stress and improve memory in people with traumatic brain injury (TBI).

Theresa Hernandez, PhD, associate chair of the department of psychology and neuroscience at the University of Colorado at Boulder, studied 38 people who had suffered a mild to moderate brain injury. Half had a type of acupressure called Jin Shin for 40 minutes twice weekly for 4 weeks; the other half had placebo acupressure. At the end of the study, which was published in the *Journal of Neurotrauma*, the people who received acupressure had better memory and attention and less stress and anxiety.

KEY BENEFITS
- Reduces stress
- Improves memory

Acupressure appears to produce what Dr. Hernandez calls stress resilience. That's crucial for these patients because a bout of stress can cause a setback. What's nice about acupressure is that it's so easy to learn that a patient can self-treat or have a family member perform it.

What It Means for You

Jin Shin practitioner Christine Palafox, who worked on the Colorado study, recommends finding leads for acupressure practitioners by contacting massage schools or medical centers.

YOGA
Learn heart-healthy poses.

Currently, the roughly 2.2 million Americans with atrial fibrillation (characterized by a quick, irregular heartbeat) have one of two treatment options: They can take medication, which can have side effects and may become less effective over time, or—if they're candidates for surgery—they can have their heart shocked electrically to regain a normal rhythm.

But now A-fib patients may have an additional choice: yoga. In research presented recently at the American College of Cardiology Scientific Session, hour-long Iyengar yoga sessions (the type that uses props like yoga blocks) done three times a week—with 15 minutes earmarked for relaxation and deep breathing—for 3 months slashed the number of A-fib episodes people had by nearly 45 percent. More astounding, during the study, 22 percent of the patients who did the prescribed amount of yoga had no A-fib episodes at all, reports cardiologist Dhanunjaya Lakkireddy, MD, director of the Center for Excellence in Atrial Fibrillation at the University of Kansas Hospital in Kansas City. Plus, the patients reported that they were also less anxious and depressed and had an improved quality of life.

KEY BENEFITS
• Regulates heartbeat
• Lowers stress

Yoga might decrease sudden surges in the autonomic nervous system, which controls heart rate, respiration, and other functions, preventing A-fib triggers.

"While we don't know enough yet to suggest that yoga replace medication, it's a good complementary treatment," says Dr. Lakkireddy.

What It Means for You

Yoga's health benefits are well established. It can help you lower stress and anxiety, battle fatigue, and improve balance. But this study reveals its perhaps most pointed effect. If you have atrial fibrillation and medicine doesn't help, or if you want to avoid surgery or simply prefer to follow a more natural treatment, practice yoga (any type is fine) a minimum of 45 minutes, three times a week.

"If you can do it daily, that's fantastic," says Dr. Lakkireddy.

MASSAGE
Try the magic of touch.

A pill that eases pain, boosts immunity, and improves mood might take many years and millions of dollars to develop, test, and market. But you don't have to wait in order to get that bevy of benefits, according to new research. Studies done at Cedars-Sinai Medical Center in Los Angeles and at the Group Health Research Institute in Seattle showed that massage already provides them. After analyzing blood samples taken from subjects pre- and post-massage, Mark H. Rapaport, MD, leader of the Cedars-Sinai study, found that a 45-minute Swedish massage brought on a major spike in lymphocytes, white blood cells that fight bacteria and viruses. It also decreased substances that cause inflammation and trigger allergies and asthma, and it lessened production of a hormone that is associated with stress levels.

"Massage helps you stay healthier," says Dr. Rapaport, now chairman of the department of psychiatry and behavioral sciences at Emory University School of Medicine in Atlanta.

KEY BENEFITS
- Eases back pain
- Boosts immunity
- Cuts stress

The Seattle study found that massage does a very good job of relieving back pain as well. It compared the benefits of two types of massage with whatever the participants were already doing, including taking medication. At the end of the study, up to 39 percent of those who got a massage said their back pain was better or gone, compared with just 4 percent of people who followed their usual care.

"For lower-back pain, massage and other treatments such as acupuncture are every bit as effective as—and sometimes more effective than—conventional medical treatments and often have less serious side effects," says senior investigator Daniel C. Cherkin, PhD.

What It Means for You

If you suffer from back pain, it's time to start taking massage seriously. Getting a weekly rubdown might relieve your discomfort, and it might also keep you healthier overall, because nagging pain can make you depressed and weaken your immune system. Some insurance plans pay for massages for cancer patients or people with musculoskeletal problems. Dr. Rapaport's findings could pave the way for research that will one day convince insurers to cover routine massages. For now, schedule a massage as often as your wallet permits.

"I get a massage once a week," Dr. Rapaport says. "It has relieved my stress. Also, I have a very bad back, and it has certainly helped that."

MEDITATION
Take a path to pain-free living.

Some 116 million Americans suffer from chronic pain, and millions more live with the debilitating symptoms of irritable bowel syndrome (IBS). Traditional treatments bring too-few lasting results. But two studies point to a surprising new path to relief: the practice of mindfulness meditation.

Mindfulness meditation operates on a simple principle. "You focus on being in the present, not on your worries," says Susan A. Gaylord, PhD, director of the mindfulness-based stress and pain management program at the University of North Carolina at Chapel Hill, who led the IBS study, which was published in the *American Journal of Gastroenterology*. When the women she studied applied mindfulness meditation to the diet and lifestyle strategies they were already using to control their IBS, the severity of their symptoms was slashed by 26 percent.

KEY BENEFITS
• Improves focus
• Cuts stress
• Reduces pain

In a recent study published in the *Journal of Neuroscience*, mindfulness meditation had equally dramatic effects on reducing pain. Researchers at Wake Forest School of Medicine found that it cut pain intensity by 40 percent—in some people, by up to 70 percent!—compared with about 25 percent for morphine and other pain relievers.

I was surprised by the dramatic results, says study leader Fadel Zeidan, PhD.

What It Means for You

To use mindfulness meditation to get relief from pain, you need to devote just 20 to 30 minutes a day to it, says Dr. Zeidan. To learn the technique, check hospitals or academic medical centers for classes.

ACUPUNCTURE
An end to pain?

Postmenopausal women with breast cancer have been prescribed aromatase inhibitors (AIs) to help prevent recurrence. But these lifesaving drugs have side effects—including joint pain—so extreme that half of women simply stop taking them. So it will be welcome news to many that acupuncture significantly reduces the pain of AI treatment.

The promise of acupuncture was driven home by a study, done at Columbia University Medical Center and published recently in the *Journal of Clinical Oncology*, that found that women on AIs who had acupuncture twice a week for 6 weeks experienced up to a 70 percent decrease in their pain, compared with those who received sham acupuncture; 20 percent felt so much better, they stopped painkillers.

"Acupuncture may interfere with pain pathways," says Dawn Hershman, MD, lead author and codirector of the breast cancer program at the Herbert Irving Comprehensive Cancer Center in New York City. "Our hope is to prove acupuncture is truly effective for AI joint pain so we can influence insurers to pay for it."

KEY BENEFITS
• Cuts pain

Virginia Ginsburg, 35, of Santa Monica, California, didn't put much stock in acupuncture for serious conditions. So when she woke up one morning in September 2009 with pain in her back and leg so excruciating that she could barely walk, she begged her husband to take her to the emergency room. She was diagnosed with sciatica, given a shot of morphine and some pain pills, and sent limping home. But after a few days, when the pain hadn't abated, she remembered how acupuncture had eased her morning sickness when she was pregnant.

"I was skeptical that it could help with a more serious condition, but I didn't know where else to turn," she says. So she called the acupuncturist again.

The results astonished her. After just one treatment, the agony began to subside. She went to two or three sessions a week, and after 10 weeks, she was completely pain free.

Stories like Ginsburg's have become increasingly common over the past few years. Marilyn Burack, 52, of Livingston, New Jersey, says she was cured of vertigo in two sessions of acupuncture after 6 months of medications had failed her. Rhalee Hughes, 38, of New York City, found that just one treatment could stop a flare-up of the pinched nerve in her neck. And similar accounts are told by many of the more than 3 million Americans who have turned to the 2,500-year-old Asian technique to relieve osteoarthritis, back pain, migraines, nausea, hot flashes, anxiety, addiction, insomnia, and infertility.

Western doctors are taking notice.

"More people in the medical community are embracing acupuncture because they see it works—often in cases where conventional medicine hasn't been as effective," says Geovanni Espinosa, ND, the director of the Integrative

Urology Center at New York University Langone Medical Center in New York City. An estimated 1,500 US physicians are now trained in acupuncture. And some hospitals even have acupuncturists on staff, who tote their needle kits into cancer and orthopedic wards.

What's behind this wave of acceptance is more than treatment trendiness. As reports of acupuncture's potency accumulate, researchers have discovered more evidence about how the technique functions—and the conditions for which it's most effective.

Does It Work?

Licensed acupuncturists point to a 2,500-year history as confirmation that the practice works. The concept that traditionally underlies acupuncture (or needling, as it's sometimes called) is that the human body has 12 meridians along which energy—called qi (pronounced chee)—flows. When these channels are "blocked" or "unbalanced," it's thought, the result is illness and pain. To unblock and balance qi, an acupuncturist inserts needles at strategic points along the meridians and their tributaries.

For Western doctors and researchers, this explanation does not rise to the level of objective proof. As a result, "there has been an explosion of study on the bio-mechanisms of acupuncture over the past 10 years, showing complex, verifiable responses in the brain, nervous system, and connective tissue," says Arya Nielsen, PhD, senior attending acupuncturist in the department of integrative medicine at Beth Israel Medical Center in New York City. One recent review named more than 20 scientifically established benefits of acupuncture, from increasing the effects of painkilling endorphins to boosting immune function to releasing anti-inflammatories (which reduce swelling and also help healing).

The latest research focuses on the connective tissue that runs under the skin, between muscles and organs. "We suspect that this tissue may be involved in the transmission of the signal from the needle to the brain," says researcher Helene Langevin, MD, professor of neurology at the University of Vermont College of Medicine in Burlington. As it turns out, the meridians that acupuncturists use to "unblock energy" actually line up with the areas of the body where needles can most easily reach this deep connective tissue. It is possible that in ancient China, acupuncturists mapped out the meridians by palpating connective tissue situated in depressions or "channels" between muscles, she says.

Despite mounting evidence, a major area of inquiry has been whether acupuncture's effectiveness can be explained away by the placebo effect—meaning that needling works only because patients believe that it will. In tests, researchers have compared "real" acupuncture with "sham" (using toothpicks or very short needles or placing needles at "inactive" points). Many—but not all—of these studies found that both versions provide some relief, but acupuncture experts claim the studies have several flaws.

First, they argue, there's no such thing as faking acupuncture—inserting a needle, no matter where or how deeply, provokes an effect in the body. Even more significantly, one University of Michigan study used brain imaging to find that the two procedures affect brain chemistry differently. Real treatments triggered the release of pain-relieving endorphins and increased the number of endorphin receptors in the brain. In contrast, the sham therapy merely produced more endorphins—without changing receptor numbers. Finally, science has started to recognize the legitimacy of the placebo in medicine.

"Expectations, the relationship between doctors and patients, and the attention a patient is given all can improve the outcome of any treatment," says Brian Berman, MD, professor of family and community medicine and director of the University of Maryland Center for Integrative Medicine in Baltimore. "But it's only been recently that conventional doctors have acknowledged that the mind does have some power in the process of healing."

What Can It Help?

Acupuncture has been studied more and more over the past few decades. Here's what the researchers have found it to benefit.

Pain: More than a dozen studies over the past decade have shown that acupuncture is more valuable than conventional care for treating osteoarthritis of the knee and lower-back pain, says Dr. Berman. It has also been shown to reduce migraine symptoms as well as medications do.

Digestive issues: Acupuncture was acknowledged as an antidote to vomiting and nausea in 1997 by a National Institutes of Health consensus panel. "The treatment releases calming neurotransmitters, such as serotonin and dopamine, and it reduces stress hormones," says Alex Moroz, MD, an acupuncturist and director of the integrative musculoskeletal medicine program at the Rusk Institute of Rehabilitation Medicine at New York University Langone Medical Center in New York City. These neurotransmitters can quiet your nervous system and induce sleepiness but may also soothe digestion, Dr. Espinosa says. Furthermore, needling relaxes muscle contractions in the stomach, found a study from Duke University School of Medicine. There is some indication that it can also help treat heartburn.

Chemo side effects: Recent studies show that acupuncture not only relieves nausea and pain in patients going through chemotherapy but also helps ease neurological symptoms such as dizziness and prickly or tingling skin. What's more, it may improve survival outcomes by enabling patients to stick to their grueling treatments.

Acupuncture is also being used to mitigate the effects of ongoing pain, fatigue, depression, and weakened immune systems. In addition to its other healing capabilities, it sparks the release of immune-system cells and stimulates production of fibroblasts, connective tissue cells that help heal wounds.

Hot flashes: Acupuncture is thought to regulate the vasomotor system (the portion of the nervous system that controls blood vessel diameter), which affects blood pressure, heart rate, and dilation of blood vessels—all of which play a role in your body overheating. In one study, acupuncture reduced hot flashes by 50 percent, and the benefits lingered for 3 months after the acupuncture was completed.

Stress, anxiety, and mild depression: Acupuncture works to counteract the fight-or-flight stress response by releasing calming, feel-good neurotransmitters such as endorphins and reducing stress hormones like cortisol. It also improves blood circulation, which oxygenates the tissues and cycles out cortisol. These effects soothe worry and ease sadness.

But Does It Hurt?

One of acupuncture's biggest obstacles to acceptance has been how off-putting many Americans find the idea of being pierced with needles. But patients generally agree that the experience is more nurturing than it is nerve-racking.

Case in point: Susan Heinle, 53. At one time, she was on her stomach in the Maplewood, New Jersey, clinic of acupuncturist Chris Butler. She'd been suffering from symptoms of chronic Lyme disease, including pain in her hips, legs, and back, plus migraines.

Butler targeted a spot on her back with his finger and inserted a superthin, flexible needle about 1½ inches long, then deftly gave it two quick twists and a tap to "stimulate" it. He repeated the process about a dozen times on her back and legs.

Before her first session, Heinle says, "I pictured big needles, like at the doctor's office, and imagined each insertion would be horrifically painful." In reality, she let out only a few mild "ouches."

"It shouldn't be painless," explains Butler. "You should feel an achy sensation for a few seconds."

After 30 minutes, Butler removed the needles, and Heinle left feeling energized—and migraine free.

What Style Should I Try?

Acupuncture originated in China, but other Eastern countries adapted and altered the basic techniques. Here are the major distinctions.

Chinese: This tends to be the strongest strain (meaning practitioners twirl the needles more), so you're more likely to feel a mild ache where the needle is inserted.

Japanese: The needles are usually finer than those used by Chinese acupuncturists and are placed more shallowly, so there's little discomfort.

Korean: The points practitioners use can vary by nation, and Korean acupuncturists often work only on a patient's hand, using tiny needles, to spark effects throughout all parts of the body.

What It Means for You

If you want to try acupuncture, a doctor's referral or friend's recommendation is a good place to start. If you don't have either, check nccaom.org, the Web site of the National Certification Commission for Acupuncture and Oriental Medicine. Make sure to look for the following:

A state license: An acupuncturist doesn't have to be a physician but should have a license. Requirements vary by state, but include between 2,000 and 3,000 hours of training (usually a 3- to 4-year master's degree program) and a series of written exams at one of the more than 65 accredited US acupuncture schools. Note: Doctors who practice acupuncture don't have to have a state acupuncture license but are required by the American Board of Medical Acupuncture to have 300 hours of training and 2 years of clinical practice, and to pass an exam.

Specialization: Acupuncturists might have areas of expertise, such as pain management, orthopedics, urology, or neurological issues.

Reasonable rates: Costs for an hour-long session typically range from $60 to $120. An acute problem might require two or three sessions a week for a few weeks; a chronic issue, one or two sessions a week for 8 weeks or more.

While the debate rages, patients are finding real relief.

Part 2

WEIGHT-LOSS
WISDOM

CHAPTER 7

The Active Calorie Diet

Turn up the heat on weight loss by eating foods that actually burn calories while you chew. You'll blast off belly fat, curb your appetite, and drop two sizes fast.

Calories. You count them. You save them. You burn as many of them as you can. But is your strategy working? If you're like 67 percent of women who are constantly (and not so terribly successfully) trying to lose weight and keep it off, the answer is no. The reason: What you think you know about calories is simply not true.

Ever since you learned what a calorie is, you've been told that they are all alike: Whether you eat 500 calories' worth of celery stalks or crème brûlée, your body will burn or store them equally. Right? Wrong. New science shows that when it comes to weight loss, calories are nowhere near alike.

Some foods take more work to eat—and therefore burn more calories while you're digesting them. Just the act of chewing foods like fruits, vegetables, whole grains, and lean cuts of meat can increase your calorie burn by up to

30 percent! And then your stomach and intestines do their jobs. In a Japanese study, researchers found that women who ate the foods that required the most work had significantly slimmer waistlines than those who ate the softest, easiest-to-eat foods. The fiber and protein in such foods take so much effort to digest that your body doesn't absorb some of their calories.

Still other calories from sources you might never consider—that are so easy to add to your meals!—can give you an even bigger burn. Caffeine and other compounds in coffee, tea, and spices such as chiles, cinnamon, and ginger fire up your central nervous system and can boost your metabolism by as much as 12 percent.

Put these foods and drinks together, and you get the Active Calorie Diet—a smart plan that takes advantage of all the new knowledge about calories. By choosing more Active Calories and fewer Couch Potato Calories (see page 75), you'll set your fat-burning engines on high all day long so you'll lose more weight—without feeling hungry. When 15 women tried the diet, they lost up to 14 pounds and 4 inches off their waistlines in just 4 weeks!

FIRE UP YOUR MEALS

Eating requires lots of energy if you choose the right foods. These four types of Active Calories stimulate your body to burn more calories. (Bonus: They also curb your appetite.)

Chewy foods (lean meats, nuts, and whole fruits and vegetables). These calories make your body work right off the fork. To maximize the chew factor, choose food in its most whole state, for example, a tuna steak instead of canned tuna, apples instead of applesauce.

Hearty foods (fruits, vegetables, brown rice, and whole grains and cereals). In addition to being chewy, these Active Calories are packed with fiber, take up more room in your belly (compared with other foods having the same number of calories), and leave less room for second helpings.

Energizing foods (coffee, black and green tea, and dark chocolate). You can get metabolism-boosting caffeine in coffee and black tea; just be careful not to load them up with milk, cream, or sugar. Green tea doesn't have much caffeine, but it does contain catechins, which are antioxidants that raise resting metabolism by 4 percent (about 80 calories a day). Dark chocolate contains both catechins and caffeine, but stick to 1 ounce per day to limit fat and calories.

Warming foods (peppers, cinnamon, ginger, garlic, cloves, mustard, and vinegar). Dieters taking capsaicin, the chemical that gives peppers their burn, doubled their energy expenditure for several hours after eating, according to a new study from UCLA. Even mild peppers contain compounds that help erase up to 100 calories a day by binding to nerve receptors and sending total fat-burning signals to your brain. Not much of a pepper person? Cinnamon, cloves, bay leaves, and garlic help too.

POWER UP YOUR PLATE

Despite all the talk about calories, you won't be counting them on this diet plan.

You should consume all four types of Active Calories each day. You'll eat mostly Chewy and Hearty foods, plus at least one Energizing or Warming food. You can have a daily snack that contains at least one type of Active Calorie food. Healthy fats such as nut butters, avocados, and salad dressings can also help boost fat burn; just limit them to 1 tablespoon for nut butters and salad dressings and one-eighth of an avocado. And drink two glasses of water with every meal to prevent digestive problems from all the protein and fiber.

Your 5-Day Meal Plan starts on page 70. Remember that the more Active Calories you include in your diet, the more calories you'll burn and weight you'll lose.

Protein (one-quarter of your plate) boosts postmeal calorie burn by 25 to 30 percent and keeps you satisfied longer than carbs or fat. The result: You can lose nearly a pound a week without doing anything else.

Fruits and vegetables (one-half of your plate) up your calorie burn by 20 percent. They're also lower in calories and higher in fiber than other carbs, so they digest more slowly to keep you full longer. Vegetables are so rich in Active Calories that you can eat as many as you want.

Foods high in fiber (one-quarter of your plate)—whole grains, legumes, and starches such as potatoes and corn—fill you up faster and give you a bigger bump in calorie burn (10 percent) than refined carbs like white bread.

YOUR 5-DAY MEAL PLAN

DAY 1			
Breakfast	Lunch	Snacks	Dinner
6 ounces Greek yogurt with ¼ cup almonds, ½ cup berries, ⅓ cup high-fiber cereal, ¾ cup fat-free milk; coffee or tea	**Tuna sandwich:** 3-ounce can of tuna, ½ cup cannellini beans, and 1 tablespoon feta cheese on small whole wheat pita with 2 tablespoons bottled vinaigrette; ½ cup grape tomatoes; 1 orange	¼ cup wasabi-roasted soybeans with popcorn (100-calorie serving)	**Orange-Sesame Chicken** (see recipe, page 76)

DAY 2			
Breakfast	Lunch	Snacks	Dinner
1 hard-cooked egg, 1 apple with 1 tablespoon peanut butter, ¾ cup high-fiber cereal (at least 5 grams fiber), ¾ cup fat-free milk; coffee or tea	**Tropical salad:** 2 cups spinach, ½ cup cut-up mango, 3 ounces cooked chicken, 2 tablespoons nuts (any kind) with 1 tablespoon balsamic vinaigrette; 10 to 15 whole grain crackers	4 ounces vanilla Greek yogurt, blueberry Soyjoy bar	**Bean burrito:** 1 cup vegetarian refried beans or black beans, ¼ cup shredded reduced-fat Cheddar cheese, and 1 cup lettuce on corn tortilla, topped with ¼ cup salsa

DAY 3			
Breakfast	Lunch	Snacks	Dinner
½ cup oatmeal (made with ½ cup 1% milk and cinnamon to taste), ¾ cup cottage cheese with 3 tablespoons almonds, 1 banana; coffee or tea	Healthy Choice, Weight Watchers, or Lean Cuisine meal; 4 ounces Greek yogurt with cinnamon; 6 or 7 baby carrots; 1 apple	4 ounces Greek yogurt with honey (mixed with a splash of lemon juice and vanilla, if desired), 2 tablespoons slivered almonds	4 ounces (cooked weight) steak, 2 cups broccoli (sautéed with garlic), 1 sweet potato with 2 teaspoons butter; green tea

DAY 4			
Breakfast	Lunch	Snacks	Dinner
Breakfast burrito: 2 scrambled eggs, $\frac{1}{4}$ cup shredded reduced-fat Cheddar cheese, $\frac{1}{2}$ small green bell pepper, chopped, and $\frac{1}{4}$ cup salsa wrapped in 6" high-fiber tortilla; 1 orange; coffee or tea	**Black Bean Burger** (see recipe, page 77)	2 mini Babybel cheeses, 1 medium apple	4 ounces (cooked weight) fish (any kind), $\frac{1}{2}$ cup fire-roasted tomatoes and $1\frac{1}{2}$ cups green beans sautéed with 2 teaspoons olive oil and hot pepper to taste, $\frac{1}{2}$ cup brown rice; green tea

DAY 5			
Breakfast	Lunch	Snacks	Dinner
2 frozen whole wheat waffles topped with $\frac{1}{2}$ cup part-skim ricotta and 1 tablespoon fruit spread (mixed), $\frac{1}{2}$ cup berries, 1 tablespoon slivered almonds, and sprinkling of cinnamon; coffee or tea	**Fast-food meal:** Small Wendy's chili and $\frac{1}{2}$ Wendy's baked potato, plain	$\frac{1}{4}$ cup mini bocconcini (fresh mozzarella balls) and $\frac{1}{2}$ cup grape tomatoes topped with balsamic vinegar to taste	**Shrimp Scampi Linguine** (see recipe, page 73)

EAT YOUR WAY THIN

Use the flavorful, fat-fighting ingredients featured in these five recipes, and you can clean your plate and lose weight—fast!

Fuel your metabolism with the right foods, and you'll zoom down the road to lasting weight loss. There's an abundance of these multitasking foods—which contain "Active Calories"—in the following recipes. You'll enjoy making these meals—and your family will love eating them.

STEAK SANDWICHES WITH PEPPERS AND ONIONS

Makes 4 servings

½ pound flank steak, thinly sliced

2 tablespoons chopped cilantro leaves

2 cloves garlic, minced

1 red onion, thinly sliced

1 green bell pepper, thinly sliced

1 poblano or Cubanelle pepper, thinly sliced

¼ teaspoon salt

4 small whole wheat submarine rolls

4 slices reduced-fat provolone or Swiss cheese

Heat the oven to 350°F. Combine the steak, cilantro, and garlic in a medium bowl and toss to coat.

Heat a large skillet coated with cooking spray over medium-high heat. Add the steak and cook, turning twice, until the edges are lightly browned but the center is still pink, 3 to 4 minutes. Transfer to a plate.

Coat the same skillet with cooking spray and add the onion, bell pepper, poblano or Cubanelle pepper, and salt. Reduce the heat to medium and cook, stirring occasionally, until the peppers are soft, 7 to 8 minutes.

Put the rolls on a baking sheet and lay 1 cheese slice on each. Warm in the oven until the cheese melts, about 5 minutes.

Add the steak and onion-pepper mixture to the rolls and serve immediately.

PER SERVING: 367 calories, 25 g protein, 40 g carbohydrates, 13 g total fat, 6 g saturated fat, 6 g fiber, 735 mg sodium

Note: Slicing your own beef (instead of using total fat-riddled frozen shaved steaks), bulking up your sandwich with vegetables, and putting it all on a hefty whole wheat roll will give you more to chew on and boost your calorie burn.

SHRIMP SCAMPI LINGUINE

Makes 4 servings

9 ounces whole wheat linguine

1 tablespoon extra virgin olive oil

1 pound medium shrimp, peeled

4 cloves garlic, minced

½ teaspoon red-pepper flakes

1 pint cherry tomatoes, halved

½ cup dry white wine or chicken broth

Juice of 1 lemon

½ teaspoon salt

3 cups packed baby spinach leaves

¼ cup finely chopped parsley

½ cup grated Parmesan cheese

Prepare the pasta according to the package directions.

Meanwhile, heat the oil in a large skillet over medium heat. Add the shrimp, garlic, and red-pepper flakes and cook until the shrimp start to turn pink, about 2 minutes.

Add the tomatoes, wine or broth, lemon juice, and salt. Cook until the tomatoes start to soften, about 1 minute. Add the spinach and parsley and cook until the spinach wilts, about 1 minute.

Drain the pasta and add to the pan. Toss to coat and serve sprinkled with the cheese.

PER SERVING: 483 calories, 38 g protein, 50 g carbohydrates, 13 g total fat, 3 g saturated fat, 11 g fiber, 665 mg sodium

MORE WAYS TO EAT YOURSELF THIN

Here are some quick and easy switches to include more "Active Calories" in your diet.

INSTEAD OF . . .	HAVE . . .
Oatmeal with sugar	Oatmeal with cinnamon
A burger with French fries	Flank steak with baked potato
Turkey on wheat with mayo	Turkey on rye with salsa
Overripe banana	Slightly green banana
Sweet-and-sour chicken with white rice	Chicken and broccoli with brown rice
Chicken nuggets	Grilled chicken breast sandwich
Macaroni salad	Black bean or 3-bean salad
Buttermilk waffles/pancakes	Buckwheat waffles/pancakes with pears
Bagel with cream cheese	2 scrambled eggs
Diet soda	Red wine

HONEY-GLAZED PORK WITH GARLIC MASHED POTATOES AND ROASTED BROCCOLI

Makes 4 servings

½ cup apple juice

2 tablespoons honey

1 tablespoon reduced-sodium soy sauce

4 cloves garlic, minced and divided

1½ pounds pork tenderloin, trimmed

¼ teaspoon ground red pepper

4 cups broccoli florets

2 tablespoons olive oil, divided

½ teaspoon salt, divided

1½ pounds Yukon gold potatoes, peeled and quartered

½ cup reduced-fat sour cream

¼ cup chopped parsley

Heat the oven to 400°F. Combine the apple juice, honey, soy sauce, and half of the garlic in a small bowl. Sprinkle the pork with the pepper.

Toss the broccoli with 1 tablespoon of the oil on a baking sheet. Sprinkle with ¼ teaspoon of the salt.

Heat the remaining 1 tablespoon of the oil in a medium ovenproof skillet over high heat. Add the pork and cook, turning once, until browned, about 8 minutes. Remove from the heat. Pour the juice mixture over the pork and transfer to the oven along with the pan of broccoli. Bake until the pork and broccoli are done, 25 to 30 minutes.

Meanwhile, put the potatoes in a medium pot and cover with cold water. Bring to a boil over high heat and cook until tender, 20 to 25 minutes.

Leave the broccoli on the baking sheet and transfer the pork to a cutting board. Return the skillet to high heat and cook the juice mixture until a thick glaze forms, 3 to 4 minutes. Remove from the heat.

Drain the potatoes and return to the pot. Add the sour cream, parsley, the remaining ¼ teaspoon salt, and the remaining garlic. Mash until smooth.

Slice the pork and put on a serving plate. Drizzle with the glaze and serve with the mashed potatoes and broccoli.

PER SERVING: 481 calories, 42 g protein, 46 g carbohydrates, 15 g total fat, 5 g saturated fat, 7 g fiber, 560 mg sodium

COUCH POTATO CALORIES

The following foods are so easily digested that you're likely to absorb every calorie and store it as fat. Even if you don't overeat, you may still gain weight.

The Pantry Stuffers

Refined and sugary foods take zero energy to digest. Check packaged foods for added sugar that goes by other names, most ending with -ose, such as fructose, maltose, and sucrose. Also watch out for corn syrup, molasses, honey, and juice concentrate.

- Candy bars and candy
- Fruit punch or fruit juice cocktails
- Sweetened cereals
- Soda
- Sweet tea

The Imposters

Beware of processed foods that are advertised as the real thing but are anything but. There's really no meat or substance left, and they're fattened up with fillers.

- Breaded chicken patties
- Chicken nuggets
- Burgers that aren't 100 percent beef or turkey
- Veggie burgers (okay on occasion, but don't make them a frequent meal)
- Bologna
- Salami
- Hot dogs

The Binge Brigade

Once you start, you just can't stop eating these starchy, high-carb foods.

- Pasta
- White rice
- Refined bread
- Muffins
- Bagels
- French fries
- Potato chips
- Biscuits
- Cookies, pie, pastries
- Doughnuts
- Ice cream

ORANGE-SESAME CHICKEN

Makes 4 servings

²/₃ cup short-grain brown rice

¾ cup orange juice

¼ cup cider vinegar

2 tablespoons reduced-sodium soy sauce

1 tablespoon brown sugar

2 teaspoons cornstarch

2 tablespoons sesame oil, divided

1½ pounds boneless, skinless chicken breasts, thinly sliced

2 cloves garlic, minced

1 tablespoon minced fresh ginger

1 teaspoon red-pepper flakes

4 ribs celery, thinly sliced

4 carrots, thinly sliced

2 cups frozen peas, thawed

2 tablespoons toasted sesame seeds

Prepare the rice according to the package directions.

Meanwhile, combine the orange juice, vinegar, soy sauce, sugar, and cornstarch in a small bowl and whisk until smooth. Set aside.

Heat 1 tablespoon of the oil in a large skillet over medium-high heat. Add the chicken, garlic, ginger, and red-pepper flakes. Cook until the chicken begins to brown, 4 to 5 minutes. Transfer to a plate.

Add the celery, carrots, and the remaining 1 tablespoon oil to the skillet. Cook until the celery begins to soften, 2 to 3 minutes.

Return the chicken to the pan and add the peas. Reduce the heat to low and add the juice mixture.

Cook for 2 to 3 minutes, scraping up any browned bits on the bottom of the pan. Sprinkle with the sesame seeds and serve immediately with the rice.

PER SERVING: 532 calories, 45 g protein, 53 g carbohydrates, 15 g total fat, 2 g saturated fat, 8 g fiber, 625 mg sodium

BLACK BEAN BURGERS

Makes 4 servings

6 ounces mushrooms, quartered

½ red onion, quartered

½ cup packed cilantro leaves

6 tablespoons soft whole wheat bread crumbs

2 cloves garlic

1 jalapeño chile pepper, seeded

1 egg white

2 teaspoons reduced-sodium soy sauce

1 can (15 ounces) no-salt-added black beans, rinsed and drained

1 tablespoon canola oil

4 slices reduced-fat Pepper Jack cheese

4 small whole wheat sandwich rolls, toasted

4 lettuce leaves

1 small tomato, sliced

Combine the mushrooms, onion, cilantro, bread crumbs, garlic, pepper, egg white, and soy sauce in a food processor. Process until finely chopped. Add the beans and pulse until coarsely chopped (10 to 15 pulses). Divide the mixture into quarters and form into patties.

Heat the oil in a large skillet over medium heat. Brown the burgers for 3 minutes per side.

Top each burger with a slice of cheese. Cover the pan and melt the cheese, about 4 minutes.

Put the burgers on the rolls and top with the lettuce and tomato.

PER SERVING: 406 calories, 21 g protein, 56 g carbohydrates, 13 g total fat, 5 g saturated fat, 11 g fiber, 680 mg sodium

Note: Satisfy your burger craving with this tasty meatless meal that supplies nearly half of your daily fiber needs. Adding jalapeño chile pepper, onion, and garlic to the mix stokes your calorie-burning engine.

BUT WAIT, THERE'S MORE

This program was adapted from *The Active Calorie Diet* by Leslie Bonci, RD, with Selene Yeager and the editors of *Prevention*, © 2011 by Rodale Inc. For the complete program, visit activecaloriediet.com to purchase the book.

CHAPTER 8

Snack Food Nation

America has a supersized snack habit—
and our waistlines are the proof. Need help?

We do it in the car, on the train, in front of the TV, on the phone, and even in bed. For too many of us, snacking has become so automatic that our brains barely register the hand-to-mouth motion. And it's not as if we're all reaching for diet-friendly apples: A 2010 study from the University of North Carolina found that most of us eat nearly 600 calories a day—roughly a third of our food—in snacks rather than meals.

Evidence of this national snack-fest is all around us. We "prefuel" and "refuel" before, during, and after workouts, taking in far more calories than we'll ever burn on the treadmill or elliptical trainer. Kids snack in the morning at school, again when they get home, and during halftime at their soccer, lacrosse, and basketball games. Even toddlers are in on the action.

Strollers come complete with compartments to hold snacks and drinks, lest the little ones go hungry for more than 5 minutes. As a result, snack foods have grown into a huge industry, totaling $64 billion a year in sales.

As if we didn't already have enough snack opportunities, chain restaurants are beefing up their so-called snack menus, which are designed to draw in customers during off-hours. Since 2007, the number of restaurant items listed as "snacks," "snackable," or "snackers" has grown by 170 percent, including items such as KFC's Snacker with a crispy chicken strip, McDonald's Angus Mushroom Swiss Snack Wrap, and the Cheese and Tomato Deep Dish Pizza from the Snack Hours Menu at Uno Chicago Grill—weighing in at 290, 430, and 830 calories, respectively.

Is it any wonder our collective waistlines have ballooned so much in just a few generations?

"In 1960, a candy bar was a treat that you saved up to buy," says Brian Wansink, PhD, professor of applied economics and management at Cornell University and the author of *Mindless Eating*. In those days, a mere twinge of hunger was not regarded as a reason to indulge. Hunger is a natural state, just like being tired, sad, or cranky. While it's not pleasant, it's not an emergency either. Think back to when you were a child and asked your mother for a snack before dinner. She didn't treat it as if it were some kind of crisis. She simply said no, warned you against "spoiling your appetite," and told you to go outside and play.

So what happened? Beginning in the 1970s, personal income increased—while government policies lowered the price of key snack-food ingredients such as high fructose corn syrup. Manufacturers hired food scientists, who fueled

SEVEN SNACKS UNDER 100 CALORIES

Here are some of our favorite hit-the-spot-without-then-needing-to-hit-the-gym snacks.

- 2 (6") corn tortillas + 2 tablespoons salsa
- 1 cup pineapple chunks + 2 teaspoons shredded coconut
- 25 pistachios
- ½ cup Cheerios + ½ cup fat-free milk
- 4 ounces honey Greek-style yogurt
- A handful (⅛ cup) of dry-roasted pumpkin seeds
- 5 fresh apricots

the trend by learning what tastes consumers found irresistible, even addictive (namely, sugar, salt, and fat). Then they figured out how to pack those flavors into betcha-can't-eat-just-one combinations. On top of it all, business schools began to churn out a new breed of executive, the brand manager, who was trained to market products aggressively as fun, exciting, and even good for boosting your energy.

"The business plan of the modern food company has been to put their foods on every street corner, making it socially acceptable to eat 24-7," explains David Kessler, MD, former commissioner of the FDA and the author of *The End of Overeating*.

The result has been a nutritional disaster. In their natural state, whole foods may be high in fat or sugar, but they're rarely high in both. Today, we have man-made snack foods with a tantalizing combination of fat and sugar rolled into one.

"Foods have become so 'hyperpalatable' that they're now capable of hijacking our brains the same way that nicotine and alcohol do," says Ashley Gearhardt, the lead author of a Yale University study on food addiction.

With all these forces arrayed against you, how can you resist? We at *Prevention* have identified some of women's biggest weaknesses—and surveyed the experts for help. Here are the most common snack traps—and our smart and healthy snacking strategies.

YOU'RE GOOD ALL DAY, BUT PIG OUT AT NIGHT

You're the Jekyll and Hyde of snacking—restricting calories so much by day that by night you're ravenous. After dinner, you trek back and forth to the fridge. Before you know it, you're cuddled up on the couch with a sleeve of Oreos.

→**Fix It!** Start with a breakfast that's really satisfying—like steel-cut oats, eggs, or Greek-style yogurt. Then at lunch, combine healthy carbs, protein, and fat. And truly savor your treats. Dean Ornish, MD, the author of *The Spectrum*, does a "chocolate meditation." Take a single piece of the best chocolate you can find and let it dissolve slowly in your mouth, paying attention to the complex flavors. You'll get more pleasure with fewer calories.

YOU STUFF YOUR FACE BEFORE DINNER

You're ravenous by the time you get home from work (join the club). You inhale whatever you get your hands on, whether it's healthy or not.

→ **Fix It!** "Planning is key," says Patricia Bannan, RD, the author of *Eat Right When Time Is Tight*, in Los Angeles. Before you get home, eat something light and nourishing to tide you over. If you're starving while you cook, munch on raw veggies such as sugar snap peas. Set yourself up for success by planning meals you can cook quickly, such as frozen veggies with a rotisserie chicken and microwaveable brown rice.

YOU CAN'T STOP EATING IN THE CAR

If you feel like you live in your car, you probably consume a lot of calories there too. Maybe you wolf down snacks straight out of the bag, with little idea of how much you've inhaled, or you pull into the nearest drive-thru for a shake or an order of fries.

→ **Fix It!** Preempt unrestrained noshing by packing portable, calorie-controlled nibbles such as small bags of cashews or an apple. Even half of a PB&J on whole wheat will do the trick. And if those fries are still calling out to you, "drive home via another route so you won't pass your favorite fast-food restaurants," says Janna L. Fikkan, PhD, a health psychologist at Duke Integrative Medicine in Durham, North Carolina. "It doesn't have to be the shortest way home, as long as you avoid the drive-thru."

YOU WORK AT HOME

It's just you and the fridge—and nobody watching. Because you have no meetings or structured activities, you can check the mail, toss in a load of laundry, play with the dog—and grab a snack (or two or four).

→ **Fix It!** Keep a log of your daily activities, including every time you get up to eat. Chances are, once you see how often you're indulging, you'll be shamed into cutting back. If you still feel the need to snack, eat at the kitchen table—and don't do anything else. Without the distraction of the computer, newspaper, or TV, you'll be much more aware of how often you eat out of habit rather than out of hunger.

YOU GRAZE AT THE OFFICE

Between the office candy bowl, the vending machine, and a co-worker's home-made brownies, your office probably stocks more snacks than a 7-Eleven. And since you're only nibbling, the calories don't count, right?

➜ **Fix It!** Launch a counteroffensive by bringing in healthy snacks—say, tamari-roasted almonds or dark chocolate—that you actually prefer over the junk. Knowing that these treats are tucked away will give you the strength to resist the disastrous jelly doughnuts. If you know ahead of time that you won't be able to leave your desk at noon, brown-bag it for lunch. With healthy fare within arm's reach, you won't need to raid your colleague's candy jar.

YOUR KIDS' SNACK HABITS ARE CONTAGIOUS

It's the diet dilemma of nearly every mom. The kids badger you into buying them sugary snacks, and then you eat them. Before you know it, you're helping with homework and munching on a Pop-Tart or a snack-size package of cookies.

➜**Fix It!** Ditch the kiddie foods, says Barbara Rolls, PhD, the author of *The Volumetrics Eating Plan*. These highly processed foods are digested in no time, leaving you wanting more. "Family-friendly snacks should include low-calorie foods that are high in water or fiber and aren't loaded with fat," she says. Try no-fuss fruits like grapes or berries—or fix some air-popped popcorn sprinkled with a bit of Parmesan.

CHAPTER 9

4 Weeks to Fit and Fabulous

*Crank up your body's fat-burning power—
even while you snooze—with this cutting-edge
plan to drop 10 pounds this month!*

Want to go from flab to fab? That's what 43-year-old Kim Hampsey and 18 other women did when they tried this revolutionary workout (and when they followed a healthy eating plan). These women lost up to 11 pounds and 8 inches in just 4 weeks. Hampsey kept it up for 8 more weeks and shed a total of 20 pounds. After shunning swimsuits for about 20 years, she's ready to wear one!

The key to this unique plan, developed with Fabio Comana, an exercise physiologist with the American Council on Exercise, is its one-two punch. Part 1 trains your body to burn more fat—even when you're sleeping—while Part 2 revs up your calorie burn for faster weight loss.

So let's get started. By following this plan, you could be shopping for smaller sizes by the end of the month!

TURN UP YOUR FAT-BURN PLAN

You'll do each of these high-powered workouts 2 days a week: fat-burning cardio intervals and metabolism-revving strength circuits.

Here's a sample weekly schedule. You can move the workouts to different days, but don't do both workouts on the same day, and don't do the same routine on back-to-back days.

DAY 1	DAY 2	DAY 3	DAY 4	DAY 5	DAY 6	DAY 7
Cardio intervals	Rest	Strength circuit	Rest	Cardio intervals	Rest	Strength circuit

FAT-BURNING CARDIO INTERVALS

Do these twice a week. Choose from the following cardio activities.

- Running

- Cycling

- Swimming

- Walking

Fat is one of two key sources of fuel your body relies on for energy; the other is glucose (stored carbs). Most of us burn about equal amounts of each when we're sleeping or sitting around. But the fitter you are, the more fat you burn at rest—up to 70 percent.

You can rev your fat-burning power by raising your ventilatory threshold 1 (VT1), the point at which you're exercising hard enough that your body shifts from using primarily fat for energy to using primarily glucose. To do this, you need to work out just past this point—a bit out of your comfort zone but not so hard that you're gasping for air (that's closer to your VT2, when you're burning almost all glucose).

Here's how it works: Warm up for 3 minutes at an easy pace. (You can carry on a conversation.) Next, pick up the intensity for a hard VT1 interval. (You should be breathing hard but able to speak in short sentences.) Recover at a moderate intensity. (You should be breathing normally and be able to speak in full sentences.) Repeat hard/recovery intervals 3 times, as shown here. Cool down for 2 minutes at an easy intensity.

WEEK 1	WEEK 2	WEEK 3	WEEK 4
3 minutes hard/ 4 minutes recovery	4 minutes hard/ 4 minutes recovery	5 minutes hard/ 5 minutes recovery	5 minutes hard/ 3 minutes recovery

METABOLISM-REVVING STRENGTH CIRCUITS

Do these moves twice a week. The routine varies a bit each week, as you'll see in the exercise descriptions that follow.

This nonstop strength routine burns about 25 percent more calories than traditional weight lifting, which usually includes longer breaks. The higher intensity can boost your metabolism for up to 38 hours postworkout.

Here's how it works: Warm up by marching in place for 3 minutes and doing

EAT TO LOSE

If you want to slim down fast, you need to pair exercise with healthy eating habits. Here's how.

Stick to about 1,600 calories a day: 300 calories for breakfast, 450 calories each for lunch and dinner, plus two 200-calorie snacks. Research shows you'll burn more calories every day by eating every 4 to 5 hours.

Drink 8 to 10 glasses of cold water daily. It takes energy for your digestive system to warm liquid to body temperature. In one study, participants burned about 50 additional calories per day by drinking 1½ liters of cold water.

Eat more magnesium-rich foods. Most of us don't consume the recommended 320 milligrams daily for women or 400 milligrams daily for men of this key nutrient that fuels muscles. Sources: spinach, black beans, ground flaxseed, scallops, tuna, almonds, cashews, and brown rice.

5 reps of that day's exercises without dumbbells. Then pick up your weights and do 10 to 12 reps (unless otherwise noted) of each exercise in the order given, taking a 15-second rest between moves. That's 1 circuit. Do 2 or 3 circuits, resting for a minute after each. For best results, always engage your core muscles to stabilize your torso before beginning each exercise.

Fit tip: You should use dumbbells that are very challenging to lift as you do the final reps of each exercise. If you feel as if you could do more than the recommended number of reps, you need a heavier weight. The amount of weight you lift might vary, depending on the exercise.

BREAKTHROUGH BOTTLES

An essential piece of workout "equipment"? Water! We gave water bottles a workout to find five that won't slip, drip, or fail to keep their cool. All of these bottles are BPA free, dishwasher safe, freezer safe, and recyclable.

GREAT FOR WATER PURISTS: Bobble, 34 oz. ($13; waterbobble.com). This bottle filters tap water. Our tester said: "My normally metallic-tasting tap water tasted like fresh spring water."

GREAT FOR CROSS-TRAINERS: MultiDrink, 20 oz. ($15; nalgene.com). With this bottle, you can drink from a straw or screw-top spout. Our tester said: "I can use the straw when I'm running or gulp from the spout between sets."

GREAT FOR THE ECO-CONSCIOUS: Modern Glass Water Bottle, 18 oz. ($20; takeyausa.com). Wary of plastic or metal? This is made of sturdy, chemical-free glass encased in silicone. Our tester said: "The protective jacket kept this pretty bottle safe even when I dropped it."

GREAT FOR HOT-WEATHER WORKOUTS: Insulated Sport Bottle, 24 oz. ($12; polarbottle.com). In this bottle, water keeps cool in the heat. Our tester said: "The shape makes it easy to grip, and my water stayed cold, even at the beach."

GREAT FOR SIPPING SPORTS DRINKS: Purist, 26 oz. ($12; specialized.com). The best part of this bottle is it doesn't trap flavors or odors. Our tester said: "Even after an all-day bike ride, my lemon-lime drink left no aftertaste."

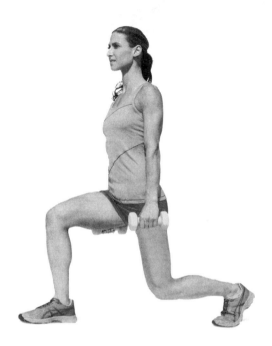

LUNGE

TONES BUTT, THIGHS

Hold the weights at your sides and stand with your right foot 2 to 3 feet in front of your left. Bend both knees 90 degrees, lowering your left knee toward the ground. Don't lean forward or back, and keep your front knee directly above your ankle. Straighten your legs to stand back up. Switch legs.

I DID IT!

"When I had to go to a black-tie event, I pulled out a dress from my closet that was a full size smaller than I usually wore. I put it on, and it looked amazing!"

—Leslie Kingston, 52, lost almost 11 pounds

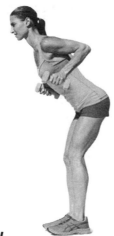

BENT-OVER ROW
TONES UPPER BACK

Hinge forward from your hips and extend your arms directly under your shoulders. Keeping your arms close to your body, bend your elbows toward the sky and pull the weights toward your ribs. Slowly straighten your arms.

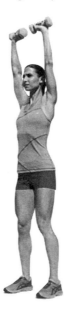

OVERHEAD PRESS
TONES SHOULDERS

Hold the weights at shoulder height with your palms facing forward. Keeping your shoulders down, straighten your arms and press the weights up. Slowly lower.

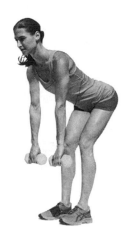

DEADLIFT
TONES BUTT, BACK OF THIGHS

Stand with your knees slightly bent. Keeping your abs tight, hinge forward from your hips, push your butt backward, and slowly lower the weights. Squeeze your glutes to stand back up.

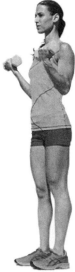

BICEPS CURL
TONES FRONT OF ARMS

Hold the weights at your sides, with your palms facing forward. Bend your elbows and curl the weights toward your shoulders, Slowly lower. Keep your elbows close to your body throughout.

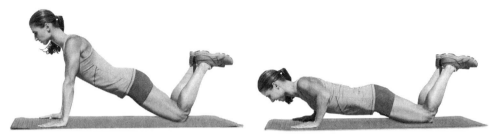

KNEELING PUSHUP
TONES CHEST, ARMS, ABS

With your hands under your shoulders, bend your elbows out to the sides and slowly lower. Don't let your hips sag toward the floor. Press back up.

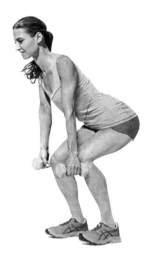

SQUAT
TONES THIGHS, BUTT

Bend your hips and push your butt backward, and then bend your knees as if you're sitting back into a chair. Keep your body weight on your heels, and your knees behind your toes. Stand back up.

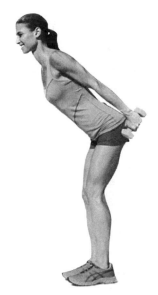

TRICEPS KICKBACK
TONES BACKS OF ARMS

Hinge forward at yourhips. Hold the weights, with your arms bent 90 degrees, and your elbows at your sides. Straighten your arms, pressing the weights back. Keep your upper arms still. Bend your elbows back to the starting position.

This week, base moves are combined to work more muscles simultaneously for a higher calorie burn.

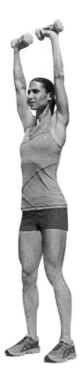

DEADLIFT PRESS
TONES BUTT, BACK OF THIGHS, SHOULDERS

Do a deadlift, and then raise your arms to shoulder height and do an overhead press. Lower your arms to your thighs and repeat the deadlift/press combo.

I DID IT!

"I used to feel stiff bending over to put my pants on. Now I feel younger when I wake up in the morning."

—Pam Garin, 49, lost nearly 9 pounds, plus 1 inch off her hips

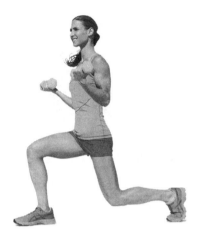

LUNGE WITH CURL
TONES FRONT OF THIGHS, BUTT, FRONT OF ARMS

Step forward and lower yourself into a lunge. Do a biceps curl. Then push off your front foot to stand back up, with your feet together. Repeat, alternating your legs each time.

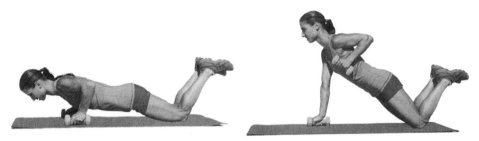

PUSHUP ROW
TONES CHEST, BACK OF ARMS, CORE, UPPER BACK

Do 10 kneeling pushups with your hands wrapped around weights on the ground. Then, staying in the "up" position, perform 8 to 10 rows with your left hand, holding the weight. Finish by doing 8 to 10 rows with your right hand.

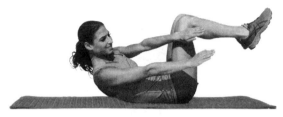

CRUNCH
TONES FRONT AND SIDES OF ABS

Lie faceup, with your arms at your sides, and your legs bent and lifted. Raise your head, neck, and shoulders, reaching your hands toward your feet. Do 15 to 20 reps. Lower your upper body for 1 count, and then reach your hands toward the outside of your right leg. Do 15 to 20 reps. Repeat, reaching toward the outside of your left leg.

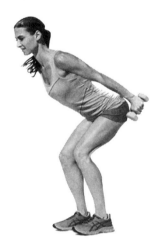

KICKBACK SQUAT
TONES FRONT OF THIGHS, BUTT, BACK OF ARMS

Stand with your arms bent at your sides. As you lower into a squat, press the weights back for a kickback, and then bend your arms as you stand back up.

This week, add balance challenges to strengthen and tone your core.

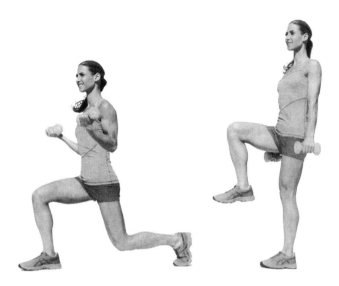

LUNGE WITH CURL AND KNEE LIFT
TONES FRONT OF THIGHS, BUTT, FRONT OF ARMS

Do a lunge with a curl. As you push off with your front foot to stand back up, raise that knee in front of you before placing your foot on the ground. Repeat, alternating legs each time.

I DID IT!

"I used to be gasping when I jogged in the park, and now I can breathe a lot easier."

—Laura Goldy, 49, lost nearly 6 pounds, plus 2 inches off her waist

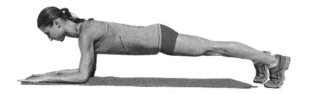

PLANK
TONES ABS

Lie facedown on the ground with your elbows under your shoulders, your forearms on the floor, your fingers pointing forward, your legs extended behind you, and your feet about hip-distance apart. Lift your hips, forming a straight line from your head to your heels, keeping your abs tight. Hold for 15 seconds, working up to 60 seconds as you get stronger. Do once.

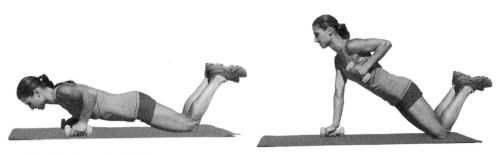

PUSHUP ROW
TONES CHEST, BACK OF ARMS, CORE, UPPER BACK

Do 10 kneeling pushups with your hands wrapped around weights on the ground. Then, staying in the "up" position, perform 8 to 10 rows with your left hand, holding a weight. Finish by doing 8 to 10 rows with your right hand.

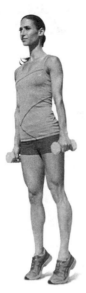

KICKBACK SQUAT WITH HEEL LIFT
TONES FRONT OF THIGHS, BUTT, BACK OF ARMS, CALVES

Do a kickback squat. Then raise your heels, coming onto the balls of your feet and your toes. Slowly lower your heels. Repeat the squat/kickback/heel-lift combo.

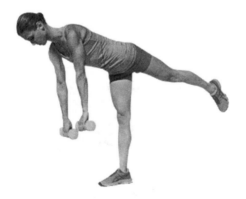

SINGLE-LEG DEADLIFT PRESS
TONES BACK OF THIGHS, BUTT, SHOULDERS

Do a deadlift balancing on your right foot, letting your left leg rise behind you. Stand back up, then do an overhead press. Do 6 to 8 reps with each leg.

This week, add some jumps to activate fast-twitch muscle fibers and rev your metabolism.

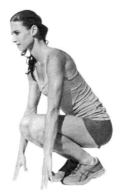

BURPEE
TONES ARMS, CHEST, ABS, BACK, FRONT OF THIGHS, BUTT

Do a kneeling pushup. Extend your legs so you're up on your toes. Jump your feet to your hands; stand. Squat and put your hands on the ground. Jump feet back and repeat. Do 3 to 5 reps.

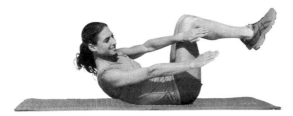

CRUNCH
TONES FRONT AND SIDES OF ABS

Lie faceup, with your arms at your sides and your legs bent and lifted. Raise your head, neck, and shoulders, reaching your hands toward your feet. Do 15 to 20 reps. Lower your upper body for 1 count, and then reach your hands toward the outside of your right leg. Do 15 to 20 reps. Repeat, reaching toward the outside of your left leg.

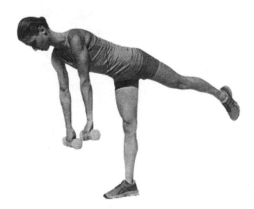

SINGLE-LEG DEADLIFT PRESS
TONES BACK OF THIGHS, BUTT, SHOULDERS

Do a deadlift balancing on your right foot, letting your left leg rise behind you. Stand back up, and then do an overhead press. Do 6 to 8 reps with each leg.

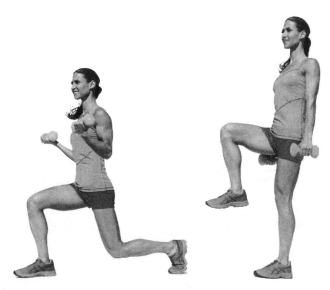

LUNGE WITH CURL AND KNEE LIFT
TONES FRONT OF THIGHS, BUTT, FRONT OF ARMS

Do a lunge with a curl. As you push off with your front foot to stand, raise that knee in front of you before placing your foot on the ground. Repeat, alternating legs each time.

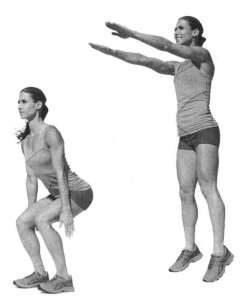

JUMP SQUAT
TONES THIGHS, BUTT, ABS, BACK

Do a squat without weights. Instead of standing back up, jump up, swinging your arms forward, and land back in a squat. Do 6 to 8 reps.

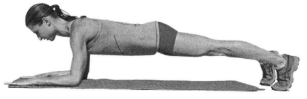

PLANK
TONES ABS

Lie facedown on the ground with your elbows under your shoulders, your forearms on the floor, your fingers pointing forward, your legs extended behind you, and your feet about hip-distance apart. Lift your hips, forming a straight line from your head to your heels, keeping your abs tight. Hold for 15 seconds, working up to 60 seconds as you get stronger. Do once.

LIQUID ASSETS

A sports drink won't make you run faster or jump higher. It'll merely replenish fluids and nutrients you lose while sweating. But there are beverages that really do have a training effect. Sip water as you work out (dehydration can slow you down), and try these other drinks for real results.

Cherry Juice

HOW MUCH: 2½ cups

BEST TIME TO SIP: Every day for a week leading up to (as well as the day of) any athletic event like a race

BEVERAGE BENEFITS: Endurance athletes who drank cherry juice before running a marathon felt less pain afterward than those who didn't. Phytochemicals in the drink appear to ease inflammation.

Fat-Free Milk

HOW MUCH: 2 to 4 cups

BEST TIME TO SIP: Right after strength training

BEVERAGE BENEFITS: The protein in the milk helps repair muscles you've exerted. The calcium and vitamin D strengthen bones and might help you lose more fat.

Green Tea

HOW MUCH: 3 to 4 cups

BEST TIME TO SIP: Daily, including right before a workout

BEVERAGE BENEFITS: The caffeine in green tea will help you work out longer. You'll also shed more fat, thanks to compounds called catechins, which increase fat burn.

Ginger Lemonade

HOW MUCH: Add ½ teaspoon grated ginger to 8 ounces of lemonade

BEST TIME TO SIP: Daily

BEVERAGE BENEFITS: Ginger, which contains anti-inflammatory compounds, has been found to ease postworkout muscle soreness by up to 25 percent.

CHAPTER 10

If Your Diet Pill Works, It's Bad for You

Leading doctors warn that the Wild West of online weight loss supplements is an increasingly risky place. Here's what you must know to protect yourself.

If you wanted to lose weight a few years ago, you might have been tempted to try Slimming Beauty Bitter Orange Slimming Capsules, a weight loss dietary supplement sold on the Internet. The label claimed that Slimming Beauty was "100% herbal" and "a natural vitamin and calcium" capsule for use even by children as young as 2. But the label didn't have two important warnings: first, that Slimming Beauty was illegally spiked with dangerous amounts of sibutramine, which is a powerful prescription-strength stimulant. Second, if you had tried it, you could have had a heart attack.

If the word *sibutramine* sounds familiar, that's because it's the generic name for Meridia, the prescription weight loss drug withdrawn from the market in 2010 at the FDA's request. Though the agency had approved the drug in 1997, a recent 10,000-patient, 6-year study showed that sibutramine upped the risk of nonfatal "cardiovascular events" like heart attacks and strokes by 16 percent, causing the FDA to reconsider.

The same day the FDA announced the Meridia recall, it also issued a consumer

HOW TO PROTECT YOURSELF

Caveat emptor: Let the buyer beware. Here's how to keep yourself well.

BE A CAUTIOUS CONSUMER. If, with your doctor's okay, you take a supplement such as fish oil or calcium, look for a seal on the bottle from NSF International, the United States Pharmacopeia, or ConsumerLab.com. Note that these companies are paid by supplement makers to evaluate their products for safety, purity, and ingredient list accuracy. They don't run lengthy patient trials to ensure that the product works—but at least you know it won't be adulterated.

SPEAK OUT ABOUT SIDE EFFECTS. If you've taken a supplement and experienced unexpected symptoms, the FDA urges you to report the problem to its MedWatch Safety Information and Adverse Event Reporting Program at www.fda.gov/medwatch/report.htm or by phone at 800-332-1088. Even a few such reports can help the FDA determine where to target its efforts to best effect.

SAY NO TO DIET SUPPLEMENTS. "There's no diet supplement or drug that I know of that's safe and effective long term," says Arthur Agatston, MD, a cardiologist and associate professor of medicine at the University of Miami Miller School of Medicine and *Prevention* editorial advisory board member. What's more, according to Steven Nissen, MD, a cardiologist at the Cleveland Clinic and a fellow *Prevention* advisory board member, even if you do lose weight by using a drug or supplement, research suggests that once you stop taking the product, you will gain back the weight and might be at greater risk of a heart attack or stroke. Both physicians recommend a healthy diet and regular exercise as the only sustainable way to lose weight and stay healthy.

warning against Slimming Beauty, citing several reports of serious side effects, including elevated blood pressure, headaches, vomiting, and insomnia. But unfortunately, the FDA doesn't have as much regulatory power over supplements as it does over drugs: It can't require intensive clinical trials before one of these products goes on the market, and it must run its own tests to prove that a supplement contains dangerous illegal drugs before it can try to remove it. Even then, there are so many similar products on the Internet that it's often unclear who actually manufactures a spiked supplement—as was the case with Slimming Beauty. After the FDA alert, the product vanished into cyberspace, but sibutramine—and other potentially dangerous substances—might still be lurking in other dietary supplements available to anyone with a Web browser and a credit card.

WHAT'S REALLY IN THOSE INTERNET DIET DRUGS

"Dietary supplements may represent the next big drug safety catastrophe," says Steven Nissen, MD, a cardiologist at the Cleveland Clinic and a *Prevention* advisory board member. "We don't know exactly what most supplements contain, so we don't know if they're actually safe."

More and more, weight loss products—along with supplements that purport to treat sexual dysfunction or enhance athletic performance—are being "adulterated" with potentially dangerous ingredients by their manufacturers.

"Originally, the makers would throw in something like caffeine to give you a kick," says Tod Cooperman, MD, president of ConsumerLab.com in White Plains, New York. "Now they're adding in compounds you find in prescription drugs without including that information on their labels." Some of these products—which are most often sold on the Internet so the manufacturers can evade regulators—may include versions of Meridia, Viagra, Cialis, or Levitra without consumers' knowledge.

The other thing consumers don't realize is that adulterated products can be far riskier than prescription diet pills. If you'd had a prescription for Meridia, for instance, you would have been under a doctor's care and would have been aware of how much sibutramine you were taking, as well as what side effects you might expect, because they were listed on the label. But in the virtually unregulated world of weight loss supplements, there's no way to know definitively what you're getting, how much—or what it can do to you.

In recent years, the FDA has gone after more than 70 tainted weight loss products, many with names like Slim Burn, 24 Hours Diet, and Natural Model, after finding that they had been adulterated with undeclared stimulants, diuretics, and antidepressants, often in amounts exceeding the maximum recommended dosages at which such drugs can be prescribed.

Sometimes the additives aren't legal even with a prescription. For example, one supplement targeted by the FDA contained fenproporex, which is a stimulant not approved in the United States because it can cause arrhythmia and possibly even sudden death.

In addition, these products often are not effective for the conditions for which they're advertised and may divert patients from legitimate medications, according to Dr. Nissen. If they do seem to be making a difference, that might be cause for concern too.

"If a weight loss supplement is working, it could be due to a stimulant whose safety is unproven," says Arthur Agatston, MD, a cardiologist and associate professor of medicine at the University of Miami Miller School of Medicine and a member of the *Prevention* advisory board. "Even if you lose weight, you may have unpleasant, even dangerous, cardiac side effects."

WHY THE RULES DON'T WORK

"People who are overweight or obese are desperate to lose weight and vulnerable to snake oil salesmen pitching weight loss products," says Dr. Nissen. "Sadly, action may not get taken until there is a high-profile death."

As far as the FDA knows, no one died after taking Slimming Beauty, but dangerous products often slide under the radar—until there's a disaster. Although the FDA is nominally charged with the safety of supplements, its ability to police them is limited by the size of the industry, the scope of the FDA's other duties, and the fact that the agency is not empowered to subject supplements to the same kind of scrutiny it gives to drugs—especially before they go on the market.

"The reality is that we are lacking resources in terms of authority, manpower, and money," admits Siobhan DeLancey, an FDA spokesperson. With an already tight budget, "we allocate our funds to best protect the public health, focusing on issues like foodborne illnesses that are causing serious illness and death," she explains.

The problem would be significant even if the FDA were better equipped. Expert estimates of the number of supplements range from 40,000 to nearly 75,000 products, including everything from vitamin C to items like Slimming Beauty. Supplement makers are required to register with the FDA—and the Council for Responsible Nutrition's president and CEO, Steve Mister, asserts that all legitimate ones who make safe products do—but the agency concedes that there are so many it can't keep track of them all. And makers of adulterated supplements may not register at all: "Anyone can set up a Web page and put a US address on it," DeLancey says. "This is a group of individuals that's willfully operating outside the law."

Cracking down on supplements' fraudulent and exaggerated advertising is the responsibility of the Federal Trade Commission. But again, resources are scant.

"When you have thousands of products and hundreds of thousands of advertisements, and you can look at only a dozen or so cases a year, then it is virtually an unregulated area," says Richard Cleland, an assistant director in the FTC's division of advertising practices.

Over the years, several bills have been proposed in Congress to give the FDA more power to take action against the offenders, including one introduced by Senators Orrin Hatch and Tom Harkin in 2010. So far, none has made it out of committee and been passed. Until that happens, it's up to you to keep yourself safe.

CHAPTER 11

The End of Dieting?

*In a radically new approach, obese people
are getting healthier precisely by not focusing
on their weight. Here's how.*

The pulse of tribal drumming fills the air. Jeannie Troy, 48 and 220 pounds, dances wildly, pogo-ing like a punk rocker at a Green Day concert and shaking her sweaty hair. All around her, women—whose body sizes range from average to well over 300 pounds—grin as they get their groove on.

This is what fitness looks like at Green Mountain at Fox Run, a center in Vermont for women determined to end their weight struggles. As the class breaks up, applause erupts and Troy grabs a towel. Her face is bright red and her extra-large purple T-shirt is blotched with sweat, but she's beaming.

"I've finally learned to take to heart that saying 'Dance like nobody's watching,'" she says.

Before coming to Green Mountain, Troy had spent countless days—and dollars—dieting. She isn't alone: At any given time, 53 percent of Americans are trying to slim down. So why, then, are so many of us overweight? Many experts believe it's because diets simply don't work for keeping weight off long term.

"If we had a 95 percent failure rate with a medication, it would never get approved by the FDA. Yet that's dieting's record," says Michelle May, MD, founder of Am I Hungry? Mindful Eating Workshops.

After decades of yo-yo dieting that only leaves them heavier than they were to start with, many women lose the will to work out and watch what they eat, and they begin dodging doctors who seem to blame all their problems on their weight. Some ultimately give up on dealing with health issues such as high blood pressure or elevated cholesterol, believing that without dramatic weight loss, it's useless.

BREAKING THE CYCLE

But according to a controversial new movement, it's possible to break this cycle of failed diets and poor health, even if you never end up in a pair of skinny jeans or in the safety zone of the BMI chart. It's known as Health At Every Size (HAES), and its principles are so radically simple that they can be difficult to grasp after a lifetime of trying to follow complicated plans full of rules, stages, calories, grams of fat, points, scales, and math.

The basic premise is that healthy behaviors can improve your life regardless of whether they result in weight loss. You abandon diets in favor of "intuitive eating," which means paying close attention to what you crave and how the foods you eat make you feel, as well as gradually learning to distinguish emotional hunger from the physical kind. For exercise, you identify any activity that provides enough fun that you don't need to force yourself to do it regularly. HAES also demands that you love and respect your body just as it is, whatever size it is right now. At its core, HAES is about stripping away rigid ideas about food and fitness.

For most doctors, it's still hard to believe health improvements are possible without weight loss. Wahida Karmally, DrPH, RD, director of nutrition at the Irving Institute for Clinical and Translational Research at Columbia University Medical Center in New York City, points out: "The research is very compelling that as your weight increases, your risk for several diseases increases also."

Yet a growing body of evidence suggests the HAES camp might have it right.

One study sponsored by the National Institutes of Health randomly assigned 78 women to either a HAES program or a conventional diet program. The HAES women were coached in adopting healthy food, activity, and lifestyle choices but were given no rigid rules or restrictions. They also participated in support groups, in which they dealt with issues regarding body acceptance and feelings that tied self-worth to their size. The women in the HAES program saw improvements (based on measures of blood pressure, cholesterol levels, activity levels, and depression) both at 6 months and at 2 years. The women in the dieting group lost weight and had improvements initially but went back to their old behaviors, weight, and blood measures within 2 years.

Troy, who lives in Thornton, Colorado, is a stalwart disciple. She calls herself a "roundy girl." ("I'm not curvy," she says. "I don't go in and out. I just go out!") Before coming to Green Mountain, she hated her body. A culinary school graduate, she worked for years in the food industry and then in the family business—a candy store. And for more than 2 decades, she was bulimic.

"I opened those bags of candy, and I stuffed down my feelings of resentment," she says quietly. Purging never caused her to lose weight. It was more about ridding herself of bad feelings than unwanted pounds.

She knew that bulimia could weaken the heart muscle, erode tooth enamel, damage the esophagus, foster stomach ulcers, and burst blood vessels in the eyes.

"But I convinced myself those things wouldn't happen to me," she says. "Then I went to the eye doctor, and the exam was taking a little longer than usual. Finally he said, 'The retina is slightly detaching.'" It was a direct result of her habitual vomiting. Her eyes fill with tears at the memory. "I thought, Oh my God, I did this to myself."

Troy realized at that moment that something had to change. Her therapist suggested she try Green Mountain; she's now on her third visit since 2008. By following the HAES practices, she's lost about 40 pounds and slashed her cholesterol by more than 100 points, from 254 in 2008 to 152 at her most recent blood test. Her triglycerides have gone from 123 to 78. She says her body composition has shifted, with more muscle and less flab. Despite her weight loss, she's still considered morbidly obese. But her cholesterol is now in the normal range, and her blood sugar indicates she isn't diabetic. Even more important, she no longer lives with a life-threatening eating disorder.

For Troy, shifting the focus from weight to health has been transformative. She's now training to be a fitness instructor, catering to other overweight and obese women—something unimaginable before she encountered HAES.

"When you're focused on weight, your whole life is consumed—pardon the pun—by what food is good or bad and what food is allowed," she says.

DO WHAT YOU LOVE; LOVE WHAT YOU DO

After Troy's last visit to Green Mountain, she went white-water rafting for the first time, and to celebrate her upcoming 50th birthday, she's planning a tandem skydive.

"I intend to do all the things I was waiting until I was thin to do," she says.

Food is now something she enjoys instead of worries about. "I still love to cook," she says. "I just made a lasagna chock-full of veggies and ground turkey." She's learned that she feels the most energized for her adventures when she eats meals made up of about half fresh vegetables, so generally that's what she has. "The more I move and the better I feel, the more I want to move and feel even

MAKE IT FUN

Who says burning calories can't be fun? Try these fusion games: Burn extra calories with fun takes on old games.

PUTTLE: In this bowling and golf hybrid, two or more players line up three pins, then putt a golf ball toward the center one. ($50; iloveputtle.com)

PICKLEBALL: To play this mash-up of badminton, tennis, and Ping-Pong, two to four players volley a Wiffle ball back and forth over a net with wooden paddles. ($97 and up; pickleballcentral.com)

ROLLORS: For this cross between bocce, bowling, and horseshoes, two to six players "bowl" wooden discs toward a small pyramid-shaped goal. ($42; rollors.net)

better," she says. "I want to make healthy meals for myself." This cycle of positive reinforcement is the opposite of the guilt-and-shame feedback loop created by years of failed diets.

Some experts believe that the negative effects of yo-yo dieting go beyond the physical and emotional tolls of being overweight or obese. According to Linda Bacon, PhD, associate nutritionist at the University of California, Davis, nutrition professor at City College of San Francisco, and author of *Health at Every Size* (the bible of the HAES movement), many studies suggest that yo-yo dieting itself increases the risk of high blood pressure, insulin resistance, and high blood cholesterol. Studies also show that a vast majority of dieting ends up being yo-yo dieting: Up to two-thirds of people who lose weight regain it within 1 year, and nearly all the rest regain it within 5 years.

Though most people understand that dieting can be destructive, it's hard to give up the dream of getting thin. Even at Green Mountain, some clients continue to calculate calories and fixate on the scale, which the staff keeps under lock and key to discourage the obsession. Some have histories of eating disorders, and many have trouble learning to respond to real hunger cues as a signal to eat, which is among the most important skills you'll need to develop if you want the HAES approach to produce results.

"Intuitive eating tunes you in to your body so you know when you're really hungry and when you've had enough," says Marsha Hudnall, RD, the program director at Green Mountain. And it's not all candy, ice cream, cheese, chips, and fries. "Some do end up eating more of those foods initially," Hudnall says. "But as you truly give yourself permission to eat what you want, you naturally gravitate to healthier choices."

Green Mountain's program does encourage women to eat more whole foods by showing them how satisfying and delicious these foods can be. Its kitchen turns out meals like walnut-pesto–encrusted Vermont-raised chicken with roasted butternut squash and arugula salad, lemon-soy grilled flank steak with garlicky mashed potatoes and lemony asparagus, and bean-and-veggie wraps with chipotle-cucumber salad and carrot bisque. There are cooking classes to teach women the skills that they need to make food like this when they return home.

Other classes help women uncover the emotional basis for many food cravings. Part of intuitive eating is realizing that sometimes you're hungry for things besides food, and there are ways other than eating to satisfy those needs.

At the end of one water aerobics class, while the other women are still panting from exertion, Rachel Peterson, 48, bellows, "I am going down that slide! Who's with me?" She quickly cheerleads several into lining up behind her. One by one they hurtle down the twisting blue chute, screaming. Peterson, an international development consultant from Leverett, Massachusetts, slides again and again and shoots up out of the turquoise water with a whoop! She has reclaimed her childhood love of the water through this program.

Before coming to Green Mountain, Peterson had been sedentary for years.

"I didn't want those wonderful-looking gym-goers to see me jiggling," she says. When she arrived at Green Mountain at 170 pounds, her knees ached—another disincentive to working out. While there, she made the connection that fitness isn't just about treadmills, weight machines, and gyms. It can be the kinds of outdoor walks and swims she truly enjoys. Today, Peterson can't believe how much better she feels, both in her bones and in her spirit.

"For the past few years, I didn't want to put on a bathing suit," she says. But here, in the pool, that self-consciousness and body shame have evaporated: "I feel like I'm six again."

Though she hasn't focused on weight loss, Peterson has dropped from a size 14 to a size 10 since her 4-week stay at Green Mountain earlier this year. She can't say how many pounds she's lost because, thanks to the HAES training she got there, she has ditched the scale.

"I have a few more inches to go before I feel like I'm in my ideal body," she says. If she does shed more weight, it won't be through dieting.

Many doctors fear that though HAES has helped people such as Troy and Peterson make important health improvements and lifestyle changes, other participants will take the movement's love-yourself-as-you-are mentality to mean it's okay to eat a half gallon of ice cream in one sitting or limit workouts to lifting the TV remote.

"We can't allow the effort to improve people's self-image to interfere with efforts to combat a serious medical concern," says David L. Katz, MD, MPH, director of Yale University's Prevention Research Center and *Prevention* advisory board member. "I agree that not everybody can be an underwear model. But when 65 percent of American adults are overweight or obese, a landslide majority is failing."

However, a growing number of professionals believe that a paradigm shift is overdue. Deb Burgard, PhD, a psychologist specializing in eating disorders who is based in the San Francisco Bay area, agrees that it's time to stop the single-minded focus on diets.

"Studies show that 'even losing a little weight helps,' but I think it's the things you do that help—the physical activity and nutrition intervention, not the weight loss itself," she says.

Even the detractors concede that if the message is articulated clearly and followed in good faith, HAES has its place for those who are determined to hop off the diet treadmill.

"If we can talk people into pursuing health, especially people who have given up on it, HAES can do a lot more good than harm," says Dr. Katz. "Besides, most people who truly focus on eating well and exercising will find that the weight eventually takes care of itself."

Bonus Weight-Loss
COOKBOOK

On the pages that follow, you'll find *Prevention*'s best recipes to help you lose weight and look great. They're delicious, nutritious, and quick and easy, too.

50 DELICIOUS RECIPES

Breakfasts

Salads and Soups

Sides

Main Dishes

Desserts

Breakfasts

MIXED FRUIT BREAKFAST SMOOTHIE

This smoothie is all-natural, tastes great, and is only about 200 calories.

Makes 1 serving

¾ cup soy milk

¼ cup low-fat ricotta cheese

½ cup frozen cranberries

⅓ cup frozen mixed fruit

Place the soy milk, cheese, cranberries, and fruit in a blender or food processor.

Process for 1 minute or until pureed and well blended.

PER SERVING: 206 calories, 12 g protein, 26 g carbohydrates, 6 g total fat, 2 g saturated fat, 5 g fiber, 150 mg sodium

PEACHY OAT BREAKFAST

When peaches are not in season, use thawed frozen peaches or canned or jarred peaches in juice, drained.

Makes 1 serving

1 cup water

¼ cup oat bran

2 tablespoons protein powder

1 teaspoon sugar

½ cup chopped fresh peaches

Ground cinnamon

Combine the water, oat bran, protein powder, and sugar in a microwaveable bowl. Stir to mix well.

Microwave on high power for about 2 minutes, checking every 30 seconds, or until thickened and the liquid is absorbed. Stir in the peaches and sprinkle with cinnamon to taste.

PER SERVING: 214 calories, 25 g protein, 32 g carbohydrates, 3 g total fat, 1 g saturated fat, 5 g fiber, 44 mg sodium

BREAKFAST PARFAITS

This nourishing breakfast is a lot of fun and refreshing on a hot morning.
Vary the fruits according to your taste and seasonal availability.

Makes 4 servings

2 cups nonfat vanilla yogurt

2 cups low-fat granola

1 cup blueberries

1 cup sliced strawberries

2 kiwifruit, chopped

Layer half of the yogurt, granola, blueberries, strawberries, and kiwifruit in 4 parfait glasses or bowls.

Repeat to fill all 4 glasses.

PER SERVING: 467 calories, 16 g protein, 68 g carbohydrates, 15 g total fat, 3 g saturated fat, 8 g fiber, 101 mg sodium

Serving Suggestions: These parfaits are perfect to serve for brunch or snacks. Assemble smaller versions in champagne glasses or custard cups.

BLUEBERRY BREAKFAST SANDWICH

If you can't find Pepperidge Farm Breakfast Bread, choose any other type of bread that contains at least 3 grams of fiber and 90 calories per slice.

Makes 1 serving

¼ cup 0% Greek yogurt

2 tablespoons pumpkin seeds

1 teaspoon honey

2 slices whole grain bread with blueberries, toasted (we used Pepperidge Farm)

½ banana, thinly sliced

Combine the yogurt, pumpkin seeds, and honey. Spread evenly over the toast.

Top 1 slice with the banana and place the other slice, spread side down, on top. Cut in half before serving.

PER SERVING: 326 calories, 14 g protein, 47 g carbohydrates, 11 g total fat, 3 g saturated fat, 6 g fiber, 274 mg sodium

BAKED GERMAN APPLE PANCAKE WITH CHERRY PRESERVES

If you don't have cherry preserves on hand, you can replace it
with strawberry jam, maple syrup, or black currant jelly.

Makes 8 servings

2 Golden Delicious apples,
cored and sliced in the food
processor

¼ cup butter, cubed

¼ cup packed brown sugar

1 cup whole milk

4 eggs

1 cup biscuit baking mix

½ teaspoon ground cinnamon

Confectioners' sugar

½ cup jarred cherry preserves

Preheat the oven to 400°F. Coat a 9" deep-dish
pie plate with cooking spray.

Place the apples, butter, and brown sugar in the
dish. Stir to combine. Cover with plastic wrap,
leaving a corner vent. Microwave on high power,
stirring once, for 6 minutes, or until partially
cooked.

Meanwhile, measure the milk in a large measuring
cup. Add the eggs. Beat with a fork until smooth.
Add the baking mix and cinnamon. Mix just until no
longer dry. Pour the batter over the apple mixture.

Bake for 30 to 35 minutes, or until puffed and
golden. Dust with confectioners' sugar. Dollop
some of the cherry preserves on each serving.

PER SERVING: 219 calories, 5 g protein, 30 g carbohydrates,
10 g total fat, 5 g saturated fat, 1 g fiber, 123 mg sodium

COCOA-ESPRESSO WAFFLES

These chocolatey treats pack a healthy wallop of fiber
and monounsaturated fats. They'll keep you smiling for hours.

Makes 5 servings

1½ cups whole grain pastry flour

½ cup unsweetened cocoa powder

2 teaspoons baking powder

¼ teaspoon baking soda

1 cup 1% milk

½ cup packed brown sugar

2 teaspoons espresso powder

3 tablespoons light olive oil

3 egg whites

⅛ teaspoon salt

2 tablespoons mini chocolate chips (optional)

Maple syrup

Whisk together the flour, cocoa powder, baking powder, and baking soda in a large bowl until combined. Make a well in the center of the flour mixture and add the milk, sugar, espresso powder, and oil. Whisk the ingredients together until blended.

Preheat a waffle iron for 4 minutes, or according to the manufacturer's instructions. (A drop of water should sizzle and bounce when dropped on the iron.) Meanwhile, beat the egg whites and salt with an electric mixer at high speed just until they form soft peaks. Fold the whites into the chocolate batter in 3 additions, folding in the chocolate chips, if desired, with the last addition of whites. Fold just until the mixture is combined.

Brush the heated waffle grids lightly with canola oil right before using. Add enough batter to almost cover the waffle grids (¾ cup) and cook for 3 to 4 minutes. Repeat with the remaining batter. (To keep warm, place a single layer of waffles on a foil-lined baking sheet in a preheated 250°F oven.) Serve with the maple syrup.

PER SERVING: 306 calories, 9 g protein, 50 g carbohydrates, 11 g total fat, 2 g saturated fat, 6 g fiber, 346 mg sodium

SPINACH AND EGGS BREAKFAST WRAPS

Makes 4 servings

4 spinach-flavored flour tortillas (12" diameter)

2 teaspoons light butter

2 cups liquid egg substitute

½ cup crumbled lemon, garlic, and herb feta cheese or ¼ cup grated Parmesan cheese

4 cups baby arugula or baby spinach

Hot-pepper sauce (optional)

Preheat a grill pan over medium-high heat. Lightly toast 1 tortilla in the pan for about 20 seconds, turn, and cook for 10 seconds longer. Set aside on a plate and cover with a slightly damp paper towel. Repeat with the remaining tortillas.

Melt the butter in a large nonstick skillet over medium heat. Pour in the egg substitute and cheese and cook, stirring, for 2 minutes. Add the greens and continue stirring, until the egg has solidified and the greens are wilted, about 1 minute longer.

Mound one quarter of the mixture on the bottom half of 1 tortilla, flap up the 2 sides, and roll to form a cylindrical package. Repeat with the remaining tortillas and filling. Cut the wraps diagonally in half and serve with hot-pepper sauce, if desired.

PER SERVING: 267 calories, 21 g protein, 34 g carbohydrates, 5 g total fat, 2 g saturated fat, 1 g fiber, 572 mg sodium

TEX-MEX BREAKFAST SANDWICH

Wake up to the flavors of the Southwest! To make sure you're helping this sandwich reach its fiber potential, read the English muffin label to ensure that whole grains are the first ingredient and that each serving offers about 100 calories.

Makes 1 serving

¼ cup liquid egg substitute

2 tablespoons shredded reduced-fat sharp Cheddar cheese

1 multigrain English muffin, toasted

2 thin slices avocado (about ½ ounce)

4 teaspoons jarred chunky salsa

Coat a small nonstick skillet with cooking spray and heat over medium-high heat. Stir in the egg substitute and cheese. Cook for 2 minutes per side.

Place the egg mixture on the bottom half of the English muffin. Top with the avocado slices and salsa, then replace the top of the muffin.

PER SERVING: 276 calories, 16 g protein, 36 g carbohydrates, 9 g total fat, 3 g saturated fat, 5 g fiber, 557 mg sodium

CHRISTMAS-BREAKFAST SAUSAGE CASSEROLE

Almost every breakfast food group is represented in this recipe: sausage, eggs, milk, bread, and cheese. The only thing missing is some fresh fruit and a cup of coffee. Instead of the ground pork sausage called for in the original recipe, you can substitute a 50%-less-fat sausage and use less of it.

Makes 6 servings

10 ounces reduced-fat turkey breakfast sausage or 50%-less-fat sausage

1 teaspoon poultry seasoning

4½ cups sourdough or other bread cubes, toasted (toast about 6 large slices and cut them into ¾" squares)

1½ cups (6 ounces) shredded reduced-fat sharp Cheddar cheese

1 teaspoon mustard powder

½ teaspoon salt (optional)

2 large eggs

4 egg whites or ½ cup liquid egg substitute

2 cups 1% milk

Crumble the sausage into a medium nonstick skillet. Cook over medium heat until nicely browned, breaking the sausage into bits as it cooks. Coat a 13" x 9" baking dish with canola oil cooking spray and set aside.

Transfer the sausage to a large bowl and add the poultry seasoning, bread cubes, cheese, mustard powder, and salt (if desired).

Combine the eggs, egg whites or substitute, and milk in the bowl of an electric mixer and beat on medium-low speed until smooth and completely blended. Drizzle the egg mixture over the sausage and bread mixture and stir to blend. Pour into the prepared baking dish, spread the top evenly, cover with foil, and chill in the refrigerator for 8 hours or overnight.

Preheat the oven to 350°F. Bake the casserole, covered, for 45 minutes. Uncover the dish, reduce the temperature to 325°F, and bake for about 20 minutes, or until set.

PER SERVING: 505 calories, 33 g protein, 63 g carbohydrates, 14 g total fat, 6 g saturated fat, 3 g fiber, 1,159 mg sodium

Salads and Soups

CHOPPED CHICKEN SALAD

Makes 4 servings

3 tablespoons red wine vinegar

2 tablespoons extra virgin olive oil

2 teaspoons Dijon mustard

¼ teaspoon salt

¼ teaspoon ground black pepper

8 cups spring mix with herbs (about 8 ounces)

4 large hard-cooked eggs, peeled and quartered

1 small cucumber, sliced

1½ cups chopped rotisserie chicken (about 8 ounces)

⅓ cup chopped red onion

Whisk together the vinegar, oil, mustard, salt, and pepper in a serving bowl.

Add the spring mix, eggs, cucumber, chicken, and onion and gently toss to combine.

Serve the salad in bowls.

PER SERVING: 276 calories, 24 g protein, 6 g carbohydrates, 17 g total fat, 4 g saturated fat, 2 g fiber, 333 mg sodium

ROASTED SQUASH SALAD

Makes 4 servings

1 butternut squash half
(1 pound), unpeeled

2 tablespoons sherry vinegar

1 tablespoon olive oil

1 tablespoon honey

2 teaspoons Dijon mustard

4 cups baby spinach

1 cup torn radicchio

$\frac{1}{4}$ cup feta cheese crumbles

3 tablespoons toasted
pumpkin seeds

Preheat the broiler.

Remove the seeds from the squash. Cut into $\frac{1}{4}$"-thick slices and put on a baking sheet lined with nonstick foil. Coat with cooking spray.

Broil the squash 5" from the heat, turning, until golden brown, about 9 minutes. Let it cool.

Whisk together the vinegar, oil, honey, and mustard in a large bowl.

Add the spinach, radicchio, cheese, and pumpkin seeds.

Toss the salad and stack it between the squash slices on 4 plates.

PER SERVING: 143 calories, 4 g protein, 21 g carbohydrates, 6 g total fat, 2 g saturated fat, 4 g fiber, 211 mg sodium

FAST AND FRESH IDEAS FOR BUTTERNUT SQUASH

Don't let its pale exterior fool you. Butternut squash has vivid orange flesh, thanks to beta-carotene. Serve butternut with a little heart-healthy fat (such as olive oil) to get the most of its cancer-fighting antioxidants. Although you can find winter squash during much of the year, they're sweetest just after the fall harvest. Choose heavy, firm, stem-on squash without soft spots; store them someplace cool and dry, and they'll keep for several weeks. Or buy this veggie peeled and cubed to save time and effort. Check the date for freshness and keep chilled.

PASTA SALAD WITH CUCUMBER, RED PEPPER, AND FETA

Put this salad together on the morning of your barbecue bash
and refrigerate until ready to serve.

Makes 4 servings

6 ounces multigrain penne, elbow, or shells pasta

½ cup fat-free sour cream

½ cup reduced-fat mayonnaise

¼ cup crumbled feta cheese

3 tablespoons chopped fresh mint leaves

3 tablespoons 2% milk

1 tablespoon Dijon mustard

1 teaspoon lemon juice

¼ teaspoon salt

¼ teaspoon ground black pepper

1 medium cucumber, chopped

1 red bell pepper, chopped

Prepare the pasta according to the package directions. Drain into a colander and rinse under cold water until cool.

Stir together the sour cream, mayonnaise, cheese, mint, milk, mustard, lemon juice, salt, and black pepper in a large bowl.

Add the pasta, cucumber, and bell pepper. Toss to coat well.

PER SERVING: 281 calories, 11 g protein, 46 g carbohydrates, 7 g total fat, 3 g saturated fat, 7 g fiber, 634 mg sodium

WALDORF APPLE SALAD

Makes 4 servings

4 small apples

3 ribs celery with leaves

1 tablespoon lemon juice

$\frac{1}{2}$ cup buttermilk

2 tablespoons cider vinegar

1 teaspoon honey

$\frac{1}{2}$ teaspoon Worcestershire sauce

Sea salt

Freshly ground black pepper

3 ounces blue cheese crumbles

$\frac{1}{3}$ cup toasted walnut pieces

Core the apples with an apple corer.

Thinly slice the apples and celery with a knife or mandoline. Toss the apples in the lemon juice.

Whisk together the buttermilk, vinegar, honey, Worcestershire sauce, salt, and pepper to taste in a small bowl.

Create 4 salad stacks, dividing apple slices, celery, blue cheese crumbles, celery leaves, and walnut pieces evenly among 4 serving plates.

Drizzle with the dressing and season with more pepper.

PER SERVING: 243 calories, 8 g protein, 27 g carbohydrates, 13 g total fat, 5 g saturated fat, 5 g fiber, 362 mg sodium

WARM POTATO SALAD WITH TARRAGON

Tarragon, scallions, and garlic add lively flavor to this potato salad.
Use dill or basil instead of the tarragon for variety.

Makes 4 servings

1½ pounds boiling potatoes

1½ tablespoons white wine vinegar

1 tablespoon Dijon mustard

½ teaspoon salt

¼ cup olive oil

1 tablespoon roughly chopped fresh tarragon

2 scallions, thinly sliced

2 cloves garlic, minced

Place the potatoes in a medium saucepan and cover with cold water. Bring to a boil over high heat. Reduce the heat to medium and cook, covered, for 20 minutes, or until tender when pierced with a fork.

Whisk together the vinegar, mustard, and salt in a medium bowl. Whisk in the oil, tarragon, scallions, and garlic.

Drain the potatoes. When cool enough to handle, cut into cubes. Add to the dressing and toss to coat well.

PER SERVING: 255 calories, 3 g protein, 31 g carbohydrates, 14 g total fat, 2 g saturated fat, 3 g fiber, 388 mg sodium

CHILLED PEA AND PESTO SOUP

Makes 4 servings

1 bag (16 ounces) frozen sweet peas

1 tablespoon finely chopped shallot

¼ cup water

¼ cup reduced-fat sour cream

3 tablespoons pesto, divided

1 cup cold water

Salt

Ground black pepper

Combine the peas, shallot, and water in a small saucepan. Cook over medium heat, stirring occasionally, until the peas are tender, about 4 minutes.

Transfer the mixture to a blender and puree with the sour cream, 5 teaspoons of the pesto, and the water.

Chill the soup for at least 2 hours and season to taste with salt and pepper.

Ladle the soup into 4 bowls and garnish each serving with 1 teaspoon of the remaining pesto.

PER SERVING: 203 calories, 9 g protein, 19 g carbohydrates, 10 g total fat, 3 g saturated fat, 6 g fiber, 267 mg sodium

CURRIED SWEET POTATO AND LENTIL SOUP

RECIPE BY MARK BITTMAN

Makes 4 servings

2 tablespoons canola oil

1 medium onion, roughly chopped

3 cloves garlic, minced

1 tablespoon minced fresh ginger

2 tablespoons curry powder

1 teaspoon salt

½ teaspoon ground black pepper

4 plum tomatoes, chopped

1 cup dried lentils

1 quart unsalted vegetable stock (we used Kitchen Basics) or water

1 can (14 ounces) light coconut milk (we used Thai Kitchen Lite) or 1½ cups stock or water

1 pound sweet potatoes, peeled and cut into ½" chunks

1 small zucchini, roughly chopped

½ cup green beans cut into thirds

½ cup chopped cilantro or fresh parsley

Heat the oil in a deep skillet or medium saucepan over medium-high heat. Add the onion and cook, stirring occasionally, until soft and translucent, about 3 minutes. Add the garlic and ginger and cook 1 minute longer. Stir in the curry powder, salt, and pepper. Cook, stirring frequently, until the powder is darkened and fragrant, 1 to 2 minutes.

Stir in the tomatoes and lentils. Add the stock and coconut milk or additional stock or water. Bring to a boil. Partially cover and reduce the heat to low so the soup bubbles gently.

Cook, stirring occasionally, until the lentils begin to soften, about 15 minutes. Stir in the potatoes and more stock or water if the mixture looks dry.

Cover and cook about 10 minutes. Stir in the zucchini and green beans, adding more water if needed to keep everything brothy. Cover and cook until the lentils and vegetables are tender, 5 to 10 minutes. Stir in the cilantro or parsley and additional salt and pepper to taste.

PER SERVING: 446 calories, 17 g protein, 63 g carbohydrates, 15 g total fat, 7 g saturated fat, 20 g fiber, 974 mg sodium

ASPARAGUS-AVOCADO SOUP

Makes 4 servings

8 ounces asparagus, cut into 1" pieces

1 avocado, chopped

1¼ cups cold water

½ cup reduced-fat sour cream, divided

2 tablespoons chopped cilantro

2 tablespoons fresh lime juice

Steam the asparagus until tender-crisp. Add to a blender with the avocado, water, half of the sour cream, the cilantro, and lime juice. Puree until smooth. Season to taste with salt and pepper.

Ladle into 4 bowls and top each with 1 tablespoon of the remaining sour cream.

PER SERVING: 112 calories, 3 g protein, 7 g carbohydrates, 9 g total fat, 3 g saturated fat, 3 g fiber, 24 mg sodium

FAST AND FRESH IDEAS FOR ASPARAGUS

Here's a case where size doesn't matter! Thick and thin asparagus are equally delicious—provided you enjoy them soon after picking. Buy bright green spears that have tightly closed tips and are uniformly thick (to ensure even cooking). Refrigerate them upright in shallow water for up to 3 days. Before cooking, snap or slice off the woody ends and peel thick stalks, if necessary, to strip away any tough skin. Asparagus supplies inulin, a special fiber that helps the "good" bacteria in your digestive tract.

PARSNIP-PEAR SOUP

Makes 4 servings

1 pound parsnips, peeled

2½ cups reduced-sodium chicken broth

½ cup water

1 Anjou pear, peeled, cored, and chopped

2 cloves garlic, smashed

¼ teaspoon garam masala + additional for garnish

½ cup 2% Greek yogurt

Cut the parsnips into 1" pieces. Simmer with the broth, water, pear (reserving some for garnish), garlic, and garam masala until tender, about 15 minutes.

Puree with the yogurt.

Garnish with the remaining pear and garam masala.

PER SERVING: 147 calories, 6 g protein, 31 g carbohydrates, 1 g total fat, 0 g saturated fat, 6 g fiber, 370 mg sodium

PICKING AND PREPARING PARSNIPS

You may think that parsnips will taste as beige as they look, but cooked until tender, this cold-weather root vegetable can be as subtly sweet as its cousin the carrot. Choose firm, medium-size parsnips without cracks (and don't confuse them with similar-looking parsley root). Refrigerate in the crisper, wrapped in paper towels and plastic, for up to 2 weeks. Peel them, and then use a sharp paring knife to remove the woody core from the larger ones before roasting, boiling, or steaming.

ROASTED VEGETABLE SOUP

This soup is creamy and earthy—and delicious.

Makes 6 servings

2 pounds carrots, peeled

½ pound parsnips, peeled

½ pound turnips, peeled

3 tablespoons olive oil, divided

1 large onion, chopped

2 tablespoons chopped fresh thyme

4 cups low-sodium chicken broth

2 cups water

Salt

Ground black pepper

Preheat the oven to 450°F.

Cut the carrots, parsnips, and turnips into 3" x ½" sticks. On a baking sheet, toss the vegetables with 1 tablespoon of the oil. Bake, stirring occasionally, for 40 minutes.

In a pot, heat the remaining 2 tablespoons oil over medium heat. Add the onion and thyme. Cook for 4 minutes. Add the roasted vegetables, broth, and water. Simmer for 15 minutes.

In a blender, puree the mixture in batches. Season to taste with salt and pepper.

PER SERVING: 168 calories, 4 g protein, 24 g carbohydrates, 7 g total fat, 1 g saturated fat, 6 g fiber, 167 mg sodium

Sides

VEGETABLE PANCAKES

These tasty vegetable pancakes will make you an "ace"
with the antioxidant vitamins A, C, and E.

Makes 4 servings

1 cup coarsely chopped
red potatoes

1 cup chopped onions

1 cup coarsely chopped
mushrooms

1 teaspoon minced garlic

½ cup shredded zucchini

½ cup shredded carrots

¼ cup all-purpose flour

2 tablespoons chopped fresh
Italian parsley

1 tablespoon chopped fresh
thyme

¼ teaspoon salt

½ teaspoon ground black
pepper

½ cup fat-free egg substitute

½ cup fresh whole wheat
bread crumbs

½ cup fat-free sour cream

½ cup mango chutney

Place the potatoes in a medium saucepan. Cover
with cold water and bring to a boil over high heat.
Reduce the heat to medium and cook for 15 to
20 minutes, or until the potatoes are tender when
tested with a sharp knife. Drain. Coat a large
nonstick skillet with cooking spray and place over
medium heat. Add the onions, mushrooms, and
garlic. Cook, stirring often, for 5 minutes, or until
the onions and mushrooms are golden. Add the
potatoes, zucchini, and carrots. Cook, stirring
often, for 3 minutes, or until the zucchini is wilted.

Add the flour, parsley, thyme, salt, and pepper.
Cook, stirring constantly, for 3 minutes. Transfer
the mixture to a large bowl and let it cool for
2 minutes. Stir in the egg substitute and bread
crumbs.

Scoop out ¼ cup of the vegetable mixture for each
pancake and shape into a ¼"-thick patty.

Wipe out the skillet and coat with cooking spray.
Place over medium heat until hot. Add the pancakes and cook for 4 to 5 minutes, or until the
bottoms are a deep golden brown. Coat the top of
the pancakes with cooking spray and turn over.
Cook for 2 to 3 minutes, or until browned.

Serve with the sour cream and chutney.

PER SERVING: 157 calories, 5 g protein, 30 g carbohydrates,
1 g total fat, 0 g saturated fat, 2 g fiber, 276 mg sodium

STUFFED ARTICHOKES

Makes 4 servings

4 large artichokes

1½ cups fresh whole wheat bread crumbs (about 3 slices)

1¼ ounces provolone cheese, chopped

¼ cup chopped parsley

3 thin slices prosciutto, finely chopped

2 tablespoons olive oil

Salt

Ground black pepper

2 cloves garlic, smashed

Heat the oven to 400°F. Remove the artichoke stems and trim 1" from the leaves. Blanch in boiling water for 5 minutes. Drain.

Scoop out the center leaves and chokes. Combine the bread crumbs, cheese, parsley, prosciutto, and oil. Spoon into the artichokes. Stand in an 8" x 8" pan. Sprinkle with the salt and pepper to taste. Add the garlic and 1 cup of water.

Cover and bake until the bottoms are tender, about 1 hour.

PER SERVING: 245 calories, 14 g protein, 27 g carbohydrates, 11 g total fat, 3 g saturated fat, 10 g fiber, 615 mg sodium

ROASTED BRUSSELS SPROUTS AND RED ONIONS

Trim and quarter the Brussels sprouts and slice the onions up to 1 day in advance. A serving of these savory sprouts supplies nearly a day's worth of vitamin C.

Makes 8 servings

1½ pounds Brussels sprouts, trimmed and quartered

1 tablespoon olive oil

1½ pounds red onions, thickly sliced

¼ cup balsamic vinegar

Sea salt

Ground black pepper

Heat the oven to 450°F. Line a large baking sheet with nonstick foil.

Spread the Brussels sprouts in a single layer in the prepared pan and toss with the oil. Roast in the upper third of the oven, stirring occasionally, for 12 minutes.

Add the onions to the pan, tossing to combine, and roast until the vegetables are tender and golden brown, about 10 minutes longer. Drizzle with the vinegar, tossing to combine, and roast 2 minutes longer. Transfer to a serving bowl and season to taste with the salt and pepper.

PER SERVING: 85 calories, 3 g protein, 15 g carbohydrates, 2 g total fat, 1 g saturated fat, 4 g fiber, 24 mg sodium

DREAMY CREAMY MACARONI AND CHEESE

Classic rich and creamy mac 'n' cheese is made healthier by using low-fat milk and reduced-fat cheese. The result: You'll never miss the fat and will love each bite of this favorite casserole. For a change of pace, try whole grain penne or rotini pasta.

Makes 4 servings

1¼ cups whole grain or low-carb elbow pasta

2 teaspoons butter or trans-free margarine

2 tablespoons all-purpose flour

2 cups 2% milk

½ teaspoon salt

⅛ teaspoon ground black pepper

Dash of hot pepper sauce (optional)

1½ cups shredded reduced-fat Cheddar cheese, divided

¼ cup whole wheat bread crumbs

Preheat the oven to 350°F. Coat a 3-quart baking dish with cooking spray.

Prepare the pasta according to the package directions (reduce the cooking time by 2 to 3 minutes). Drain.

Melt the butter in a medium saucepan over medium heat. Stir in the flour and cook, stirring constantly, for 2 minutes, or until browned. Whisk in the milk, salt, black pepper, and hot pepper sauce, if using. Cook, stirring frequently, over medium heat for 5 minutes, or until just boiling.

Add 1¼ cups of the cheese and cook, stirring constantly, for 2 minutes, or until melted.

Mix the pasta and cheese sauce and pour into the prepared baking dish. Combine the remaining ¼ cup cheese and the bread crumbs in a small bowl. Sprinkle over the casserole. Bake for 30 minutes, or until bubbling and golden brown.

PER SERVING: 289 calories, 20 g protein, 36 g carbohydrates, 8 g total fat, 5 g saturated fat, 3 g fiber, 637 mg sodium

BEANS WITH HERBED TOMATOES AND GOAT CHEESE

Makes 4 servings

3 medium tomatoes, seeded and chopped

¼ cup chopped fresh basil or 1 tablespoon dried

¼ cup chopped fresh oregano or 1 tablespoon dried

2 scallions, sliced

2 cloves garlic, minced

¼ teaspoon salt

¼ teaspoon ground black pepper

1 can (15 ounces) kidney beans, rinsed and drained

1 can (15 ounces) navy beans, rinsed and drained

1 cup crumbled semisoft goat cheese or feta cheese

Combine the tomatoes, basil, oregano, scallions, garlic, salt, and pepper in a medium bowl. Let stand at room temperature for 30 minutes to 2 hours.

Place the kidney and navy beans in a medium microwaveable bowl. Microwave on medium power for 1 to 2 minutes, stirring once. Stir the beans into the tomato mixture and sprinkle with the cheese.

PER SERVING: 276 calories, 17 g protein, 32 g carbohydrates, 10 g total fat, 6 g saturated fat, 9 g fiber, 851 mg sodium

Note: Serve this hearty fresh tomato dish with steamed fish or chicken and whole grain rolls.

BAKED MUSHROOM RISOTTO

Makes 8 servings

2 tablespoons olive oil

½ medium onion, finely chopped

½ teaspoon salt

1 pound sliced mushrooms

⅓ cup dry white wine

1½ cups Arborio rice

3 cups chicken stock (we used Kitchen Basics), heated

¾ cup grated Parmesan cheese, divided

Ground black pepper

Heat the oven to 350°F.

Heat the oil in a Dutch oven over medium-high heat. Add the onion and salt and cook until the onion begins to turn golden brown, about 7 minutes. Add the mushrooms and cook, stirring occasionally, until the liquid given off by the mushrooms evaporates and the mushrooms brown, about 15 minutes.

Add the wine and cook until evaporated, about 3 minutes. Transfer to an ovenproof serving dish if desired. Stir in the rice, stock, and ½ cup of the cheese. Bake until the rice is cooked and all the liquid is absorbed, about 35 minutes. Season to taste with salt and black pepper and top with the remaining ¼ cup cheese.

PER SERVING: 246 calories, 11 g protein, 36 g carbohydrates, 7 g total fat, 2 g saturated fat, 1 g fiber, 427 mg sodium

SWEET POTATO GRATIN WITH PECAN-CRUMB TOPPING

You can prepare the recipe through step 2, and chill the mashed sweet potatoes up to 2 days in advance. Citrus plays up the natural sweetness of these fiber-rich potatoes, so skip the marshmallows and added sugar.

Makes 8 servings

3 large sweet potatoes

2 tablespoons unsalted butter, melted

1½ teaspoons finely grated orange peel

2 tablespoons fresh lemon juice

2 tablespoons fresh orange juice

1 tablespoon minced garlic

½ teaspoon ground allspice

Sea salt

½ cup fresh whole wheat bread crumbs

⅓ cup pecan halves, coarsely chopped

¼ cup chopped scallion greens

2 tablespoons finely grated Parmesan cheese

Heat the oven to 400°F with the rack in the center position. Prick the potatoes several times with a fork and wrap each in foil.

Roast the potatoes on the oven rack until very tender, about 45 minutes. Carefully unwrap the foil and halve the potatoes. Scoop the flesh into a bowl. Mash the potatoes with the butter, orange peel, juices, garlic, allspice, and salt to taste. Set aside.

Toss together the bread crumbs, pecans, scallions, and cheese in a bowl.

Reduce the heat to 375°F and coat with cooking spray a 1-quart shallow glass pie pan or ceramic baking dish. Spoon the potatoes into the dish and top with the crumb mixture. Bake until the crumbs are golden and the potato mixture is hot, about 30 minutes.

PER SERVING: 230 calories, 5 g protein, 39 g carbohydrates, 7 g total fat, 3 g saturated fat, 6 g fiber, 98 mg sodium

MASHED POTATOES

Makes 12 servings

4 pounds Yukon gold potatoes

1 teaspoon sea salt

1 cup 2% milk, warmed

¼ cup unsalted butter

Ground black pepper

Peel and quarter the potatoes. Add to a large pot, cover with 3" of cold water, and bring to a boil.

Add the salt and simmer the potatoes until tender, about 15 minutes. Reserve 1 cup of the cooking liquid and drain the potatoes in a colander.

Return the potatoes to the pot with the milk, butter, and ½ cup of the reserved liquid. Mash with a potato masher until almost smooth, adding more cooking liquid as needed. Season to taste with additional sea salt and pepper.

PER SERVING: 173 calories, 3 g protein, 31 g carbohydrates, 5 g total fat, 3 g saturated fat, 3 g fiber, 371 mg sodium

ALTERNATES:

BACON-ONION: Mix 8 chopped, cooked slices of bacon and ¾ cup finely chopped scallion greens into the finished potatoes.

GARLIC: Wrap 1 head of garlic in foil. Roast in a 400°F oven for 45 minutes. Squeeze the cloves into the milk for the potatoes and mash with a fork.

SPICY: Fold 2 teaspoons canned chipotle in adobo sauce (or to taste) and ¼ cup reduced-fat sour cream into the finished potatoes.

EXTRA CREAMY: Whisk ½ cup reduced-fat cream cheese and ¾ cup chopped fresh chives into the finished potatoes.

BLUE CHEESE: Use low-fat buttermilk instead of milk and fold in ¾ cup of blue cheese crumbles.

HERBS: Stir fresh herbs (such as 1 cup chopped flat-leaf parsley, chives, or chervil) into the finished potatoes.

CREAMY SWEET CORN

This special low-fat version of a Louisiana recipe (which often includes cream and butter or bacon fat) still tastes luscious. In Louisiana it's called maque choux, pronounced "mock shoe."

Makes 4 servings

1 tablespoon olive oil

1 small onion, finely chopped (about ½ cup)

¼ red bell pepper, finely chopped (about ¼ cup)

1 small rib celery, finely chopped (about ¼ cup)

2 cups fresh corn kernels (from about 4 ears) or 2 cups frozen corn kernels

1 teaspoon minced garlic (1 clove)

¾ teaspoon salt

⅛ teaspoon ground red pepper

½ cup fat-free evaporated milk

Heat the oil over medium heat in a medium saucepan. Add the onion, bell pepper, and celery and cook, stirring often, until soft, about 4 minutes.

Add the corn, garlic, salt, and ground red pepper and cook for 10 minutes, stirring often.

Pour in the milk. Cook over low heat until the mixture is creamy, about 2 minutes.

PER SERVING: 132 calories, 5 g protein, 21 g carbohydrates, 4 g total fat, 1 g saturated fat, 3 g fiber, 489 mg sodium

Main Dishes

CHICKEN–SWEET POTATO STIR-FRY

Some of the big tastes in Mexican food—cumin, jalapeño, and cilantro,
as well as garlic, onion, and black pepper—contribute mouthwatering
zest to this not-so-south-of-the-border dish.

Makes 4 servings

1 cup water

½ cup quinoa, rinsed and drained

1 medium sweet potato (about 8 ounces), peeled and cut into ½" cubes

4 teaspoons canola oil, divided

12 ounces boneless, skinless chicken breast, cut into ½" pieces

1 medium onion, chopped

1 jalapeño chile pepper, finely chopped

1 medium red bell pepper, chopped

1 clove garlic, minced

1 teaspoon ground cumin

1 cup frozen peas

3 tablespoons chopped fresh cilantro

¼ teaspoon salt

⅛ teaspoon ground black pepper

Combine the water and quinoa in a small saucepan over medium-high heat. Bring to a boil, reduce the heat to medium, and simmer until the liquid has been absorbed, 12 to 15 minutes.

Meanwhile, put the sweet potato in a small saucepan with enough cold water to cover by 2". Bring to a boil over medium-high heat and cook until just tender, 3 to 4 minutes. Drain.

Heat 2 teaspoons of the oil in a large nonstick or cast-iron skillet over medium-high heat. Add the chicken and cook, stirring occasionally, until starting to brown, about 4 minutes. Transfer to a bowl and set aside.

Return the pan to the heat and add the remaining 2 teaspoons oil. Stir in the onion and jalapeño pepper. Cook, stirring occasionally, for 1 minute. Add the bell pepper, garlic, and cumin.

Cook until the vegetables start to soften, 2 to 3 minutes. Stir in the peas and the reserved chicken and cook for 2 minutes. Add the quinoa and sweet potato. Cook, stirring frequently, until heated through, 1 to 2 minutes. Remove from the heat and stir in the cilantro, salt, and black pepper.

PER SERVING: 307 calories, 24 g protein, 34 g carbohydrates, 8 g total fat, 1 g saturated fat, 6 g fiber, 264 mg sodium

CHICKEN WITH WALNUTS AND SPINACH

Makes 4 servings

⅓ cup chopped onion

1 tablespoon olive oil

1 cup walnut pieces, chopped, divided

1 cup baby spinach, chopped

½ cup grated provolone

4 thin-sliced boneless, skinless chicken breasts, seasoned with ¼ teaspoon salt and ¼ teaspoon ground black pepper

Heat the oven to 375°F.

Cook the onion in the oil in a skillet over medium-low heat for 5 minutes, or until softened. Add ½ cup of the walnuts and cook for 1 minute. Increase the heat to medium. Add the spinach. Cook until wilted, about 2 minutes.

Put the mixture in a bowl and stir in the cheese. Divide among the chicken slices and roll up to enclose. Spray the chicken with oil and roll in the remaining nuts. Bake on a greased baking sheet for 30 to 35 minutes, or until no longer pink and the juices run clear.

PER SERVING: 413 calories, 33 g protein, 6 g carbohydrates, 30 g total fat, 5 g saturated fat, 3 g fiber, 412 mg sodium

GRILLED RIB-EYE STEAK
WITH MUSTARD SAUCE

Makes 6 servings

3 tablespoons mayonnaise

1½ teaspoons sour cream or plain yogurt

1 scallion, finely chopped

1 teaspoon dry mustard

¾ teaspoon soy sauce

½ teaspoon ground black pepper, divided

¼ teaspoon salt, divided

1 boneless beef rib-eye steak (1½ pounds), 1" thick, fat trimmed

Combine the mayonnaise, sour cream or yogurt, scallion, mustard, soy sauce, ¼ teaspoon of the pepper, and ⅛ teaspoon of the salt in a small bowl. Cover and let sit at room temperature.

Meanwhile, coat a grill rack with cooking spray. Preheat the grill. Season the beef with the remaining ¼ teaspoon pepper and the remaining ⅛ teaspoon salt. Grill, turning once, until a thermometer inserted in the center registers 160°F for medium, 11 to 13 minutes. Remove to a platter and let rest for 5 minutes.

Thinly slice the steak and serve topped with the mustard sauce.

PER SERVING: 221 calories, 23 g protein, 2 g carbohydrates, 13 g total fat, 4 g saturated fat, 0 g fiber, 265 mg sodium

Note: Leftovers can be covered and refrigerated for up to 3 days. Add to grain and vegetable salads for a quick main dish. Or serve leftover slices of steak wrapped around slices of Swiss cheese, sprouts, and sliced tomatoes for a sandwich or snack. The sauce can be made ahead and refrigerated for up to 5 days.

BEEF STROGANOFF

This hearty stew is delicious served over hot cooked brown rice
or whole wheat couscous.

Makes 6 servings

1½ pounds lean beef stew meat

1 pound mushrooms, sliced

1 onion, chopped

1 clove garlic, minced

1 can (10.75 ounces) fat-free cream of mushroom soup

1 cup water

1 teaspoon salt

¼ teaspoon ground black pepper

1 cup fat-free sour cream

Coat a 4- to 6-quart slow cooker with cooking spray. Combine the beef, mushrooms, onion, garlic, soup, water, salt, and pepper in the cooker, stirring until well blended.

Cover and cook on low for 6 to 8 hours.

Stir in the sour cream. Cover and cook on high for 5 minutes, or until heated through.

PER SERVING: 285 calories, 29 g protein, 15 g carbohydrates, 12 g total fat, 5 g saturated fat, 2 g fiber, 870 mg sodium

APPLE SAUSAGE PENNE

Here's a great way to introduce moderation into your meals.
The low-carb pasta and the apples provide plenty of fiber, while the half-and-half
adds a touch of decadence. Choosing low-fat turkey sausage keeps the fat
and calories lower than if using regular sausage or kielbasa.

Makes 4 servings

2 cups low-carb penne pasta

1 pound Italian low-fat turkey sausage, diagonally cut into ¼" slices

4 Red Delicious apples, cubed

½ cup half-and-half

¼ cup crumbled low-fat Gorgonzola or other blue cheese

¼ cup chopped fresh basil

Prepare the pasta according to the package directions. Drain.

Meanwhile, stir the sausage slices in a large saucepan over medium-high heat until well browned. Add the apples and stir for 5 minutes, or until the apples are golden. Add the pasta, half-and-half, and cheese and cook for 2 minutes, stirring, until heated through. Sprinkle with the basil before serving.

PER SERVING: 566 calories, 30 g protein, 71 g carbohydrates, 20 g total fat, 4 g saturated fat, 7 g fiber, 879 mg sodium

GLAZED PORK TENDERLOIN WITH SUCCOTASH

Fresh ginger has more oomph than the dried variety. It gives a big shot
of taste to the pork, and its heat is strengthened by the black pepper.
Vinegar, onion, and herbs heighten the flavor of the succotash.

Makes 4 servings

¼ cup apricot preserves

1 tablespoon grated fresh ginger

1 pound lean pork tenderloin, trimmed of all visible fat

¼ teaspoon ground black pepper

⅛ + ¼ teaspoon salt

1 teaspoon extra virgin olive oil

1 package (10 ounces) frozen cut okra

½ medium onion, chopped

1 teaspoon dried oregano

1 cup fresh or frozen corn kernels

2 teaspoons cider vinegar

1 teaspoon sugar

3 tablespoons thinly sliced fresh basil

Heat the broiler or grill to medium-high.

Combine the preserves and ginger in a small bowl. Sprinkle the pork with the pepper and ⅛ teaspoon of the salt. Broil or grill the pork for 10 minutes, turn, and cook for 10 minutes. Brush the meat with half of the preserve mixture and continue cooking for 2 minutes. Turn and brush with the remaining mixture. Cook for 2 minutes, or until a thermometer inserted into the thickest portion registers 160°F and the juices run clear. Turn the pork and broil or grill for 30 seconds to set the glaze. Transfer to a cutting board, cover loosely with foil, and let stand for 10 minutes. Cut into 16 slices.

Meanwhile, heat the oil in a large nonstick skillet over medium-high heat. Add the okra, onion, and oregano and cook, stirring occasionally, until the onion starts to brown and the okra stops giving off liquid, 6 to 7 minutes.

Stir in the corn and cook until starting to brown slightly, about 3 minutes. Add the vinegar and sugar and cook for 1 minute. Remove from the heat and stir in the basil and the remaining ¼ teaspoon salt. Serve with the sliced pork.

PER SERVING: 251 calories, 25 g protein, 29 g carbohydrates, 5 g total fat, 1 g saturated fat, 3 g fiber, 279 mg sodium

COUSCOUS WITH CHICKPEAS, DRIED FRUIT, AND CILANTRO

Limit sodium: Perk up low-salt beans with the sweetness
of orange, apricot, and cranberry.

Makes 4 servings

½ cup water

¼ teaspoon ground allspice

1 cup orange juice, divided

½ teaspoon salt, divided

¾ cup whole wheat couscous

2 tablespoons olive oil

1 medium onion, sliced

1 medium green bell pepper, thinly sliced

3 cloves garlic, minced

1½ teaspoons curry powder

1 can (15 ounces) no-salt-added chickpeas, rinsed and drained

½ cup dried apricots, sliced

½ cup dried sweetened cranberries

3 tablespoons chopped cilantro

Combine the water, allspice, ½ cup of the orange juice, and ¼ teaspoon of the salt in a saucepan over medium-high heat. Bring to a boil, stir in the couscous, cover, remove from the heat, and let stand for 5 minutes. Fluff with a fork.

Meanwhile, heat the oil in a large nonstick skillet over medium-high heat. Add the onion, pepper, garlic, and curry powder. Cook, stirring occasionally, until the vegetables are tender, about 10 minutes. Add the chickpeas, apricots, and cranberries. Cook, stirring occasionally, for 2 minutes.

Pour in the remaining ½ cup orange juice and cook, stirring often, for 1 minute. Remove from the heat and stir in the cilantro and the remaining ¼ teaspoon salt. Serve over the couscous.

PER SERVING: 363 calories, 9 g protein, 67 g carbohydrates, 9 g total fat, 1 g saturated fat, 9 g fiber, 320 mg sodium

TORTILLA "LASAGNA"

Onion and garlic give any dish unmatchable depth of flavor, along with a big nutritional bonus. Both contain sulfur, which is good for maintaining normal blood pressure—and gives them their aromatic qualities. Onions are also full of quercetin, an antioxidant that may help protect against cancer.

Recipe by Mark Bittman

Makes 4 servings

1 teaspoon olive oil

1 onion, chopped

2 cloves garlic, chopped

1 teaspoon ground cumin

1½ cups crushed tomatoes

1 cup water

1 can (4 ounces) mild diced chiles, drained (we used fire roasted)

1 package (8 ounces) corn tortillas (6" diameter)

1¼ cups shredded Monterey Jack cheese

Heat the oven to 400°F. Coat a baking sheet with cooking spray.

Heat the oil in a large skillet over medium heat. Add the onion and garlic and cook, stirring, for about 5 minutes, or until softened. Add the cumin and cook for 1 minute.

Add the tomatoes, water, and chiles and bring to a boil over high heat. Reduce the heat to medium-low and simmer, stirring occasionally, until the sauce is thickened, about 15 minutes.

Coat 1 side of each tortilla with oil and cut into 1" strips. Put on the baking sheet. Bake until crisp, about 10 minutes. Set aside. Reduce the oven temperature to 350°F.

Layer half of the tortilla strips in a 2-quart baking dish and top with half of the sauce and cheese. Add the remaining tortilla strips, sauce, and cheese. Bake until the cheese is melted and the casserole is bubbly, about 20 minutes.

PER SERVING: 314 calories, 14 g protein, 37 g carbohydrates, 14 g total fat, 7 g saturated fat, 7 g fiber, 420 mg sodium

MEDITERRANEAN PIZZA

Being heavy-handed with sauces and toppings on a thin-crust pizza will guarantee a soggy pie. To keep it crispy, grill one side of the crust until golden brown, then turn and spread with a thin layer of sauce and a light sprinkling of your favorite flavorings.

Makes 4 servings

1 jar (3.5 ounces) roasted red peppers

¼ cup crumbled feta (1 ounce)

1 tablespoon red wine vinegar

1 cup marinated artichoke hearts

16 thin lemon slices

2 Whole Wheat Pizza Crusts (see "Make Some Dough!" on page 155)

½ cup packed fresh baby spinach leaves

8 quartered pitted kalamata olives

2 teaspoons extra virgin olive oil

Ground black pepper

Heat the grill to medium-high.

Rinse and drain the peppers and puree in a blender with the cheese and vinegar.

Rinse, drain, and halve the artichoke hearts.

Grill the artichokes and the lemon, turning, until marked, about 2 minutes. Remove from the heat.

Unwrap the pizza crusts and lightly coat 1 side of each with olive oil spray.

Place the crusts oil side down on the grill and heat until bottoms are golden, about 2 minutes. Turn the crusts and spread evenly with the blended red-pepper sauce.

Sprinkle the crusts evenly with the spinach and the olives. Scatter the artichokes and lemon evenly over top.

Grill the pizzas for 2 minutes. Remove from the heat. Top with the oil and black pepper to taste.

Cut each pizza into 4 slices.

PER 2-SLICE SERVING: 217 calories, 7 g protein, 31 g carbohydrates, 9 g total fat, 2 g saturated fat, 5 g fiber, 581 mg sodium

MAKE SOME DOUGH!

A thin whole wheat crust supplies fiber and keeps calories under control. You can make the dough, roll it out, and freeze it (wrapped tightly in plastic) for 1 month. Frozen crusts can go directly on the grill.

TIME-SAVING TRICK: With Fleishmann's Pizza Crust Yeast ($2 for a 3-pack), you can skip the 1-hour rising time and roll out the dough right after kneading.

WHOLE WHEAT PIZZA CRUSTS

Makes 2 servings per pizza

¾ cup warm water (105°–115°F)

1 package (¼ ounce) active dry yeast

½ teaspoon sugar

1 cup whole wheat flour

1 cup all-purpose flour

1½ teaspoons extra virgin olive oil

½ teaspoon kosher salt

Stir together the water, yeast, and sugar in a medium bowl. Let stand until foamy, about 10 minutes.

Stir in the whole wheat flour, all-purpose flour, oil, and salt.

On a lightly floured surface, knead the dough lightly until smooth, about 2 minutes.

Lightly oil a medium bowl. Place the dough in the bowl. Cover the bowl loosely with plastic wrap and let the dough rise until doubled in size, about 1 hour.

Form the dough into 4 balls.

Roll out a dough ball on a very lightly floured surface until ⅛" thick (about 10" diameter).

Transfer to a baking sheet lined with plastic wrap and cover tightly with another sheet of plastic. Repeat with remaining dough.

Freeze the dough until firm (about 10 minutes) or until ready to use.

PER ½ CRUST: 120 calories, 4 g protein, 23 g carbohydrates, 2 g total fat, 0 g saturated fat, 2 g fiber, 242 mg sodium

WHITE BEAN "BLT" TARTINE

Makes 4 servings

½ cup cherry tomatoes, halved

¾ cup canned great Northern beans, rinsed and drained

2 tablespoons crumbled feta

2 tablespoons chopped fresh flat-leaf parsley

1 tablespoon chopped fresh basil

¼ teaspoon chopped garlic

2 tablespoons extra virgin olive oil, divided

4 slices (¼" thick) rustic whole grain bread (about 4 ounces total), toasted

¼ cup sliced radicchio

Salt

Ground black pepper

Preheat the broiler.

Put the tomatoes cut side up on a foil-lined baking sheet. Broil 5" from the heat until wilted, about 3 minutes. Set aside.

In a food processor, puree the beans, feta, parsley, basil, garlic, and 1 tablespoon of the oil until smooth. (Makes about ⅔ cup.)

Spread the bean mixture evenly on the bread slices and top with the radicchio and roasted tomatoes. Drizzle with the remaining 1 tablespoon oil and season with salt and pepper to taste.

PER SERVING: 197 calories, 5 g protein, 23 g carbohydrates, 10 g total fat, 2 g saturated fat, 4 g fiber, 193 mg sodium

Desserts

FANCY FRUIT TART

Makes 10 servings

2 cups all-purpose or gluten-free flour

1 teaspoon baking powder

½ cup (1 stick) trans-free margarine, cut into small pieces + 2 tablespoons

½ cup agave nectar, divided

3 tablespoons milk (2% or fat-free), divided

1 large egg

1 teaspoon vanilla extract

1 package (8 ounces) fat-free cream cheese, softened

1 tablespoon lemon juice

4 cups sliced fruit or berries, such as apricots, strawberries, and blueberries

½ cup all-fruit apricot spreadable fruit

Combine the flour and baking powder in a food processor. Add the ½ cup margarine pieces and pulse until crumbs form. With the processor running, add ¼ cup of the nectar, 1 tablespoon of the milk, the egg, and vanilla, and process until the dough forms a ball. Form into a disk and wrap with plastic wrap. Chill for 3 hours.

Preheat the oven to 375°F.

Press the dough into a 12" pizza pan or a 10" tart pan. Prick all over with a fork. Bake in the pizza pan for 8 to 10 minutes, or until browned, or bake in the tart pan for 7 to 8 minutes. Cool completely on a rack.

Beat the cream cheese, the remaining 2 tablespoons margarine, the remaining ¼ cup nectar, the remaining 2 tablespoons milk, and the lemon juice with an electric mixer on medium speed until blended. Spread on the crust. Arrange the fruit over the filling.

Place the spreadable fruit in a microwaveable bowl. Microwave on high for 1 minute, stirring. Brush over the fruit.

PER SERVING: 334 calories, 7 g protein, 49 g carbohydrates, 13 g total fat, 5 g saturated fat, 2 g fiber, 307 mg sodium

Note: If you're using a pizza pan, create a "lip" around the edge of the pan to form sides.

LEMON SPONGE CAKE WITH MIXED BERRIES

This cake is healthy, easy, and utterly delicious!

Makes 12 servings

7 large egg whites (1 cup)

1 teaspoon cream of tartar

2 tablespoons + 1 cup superfine sugar

5 large egg yolks (⅓ cup)

2 tablespoons hot water

1 tablespoon freshly grated lemon peel

1 teaspoon vanilla extract

1 teaspoon baking powder

Pinch of salt

1 cup cake flour

18 ounces mixed fresh berries (about 3 cups)

¼ cup honey

2 tablespoons lemon juice

Preheat the oven to 350°F. With an electric mixer, beat the egg whites and cream of tartar in a large bowl until soft peaks form. Beat in 2 tablespoons of the sugar.

In another large bowl, combine the egg yolks and remaining 1 cup sugar. Add the hot water and beat until very pale yellow in color, about 4 minutes. Beat in the lemon peel, vanilla, baking powder, and salt. Gradually beat in the flour, then gently fold one-third of the egg whites into the yolk mixture. Gently fold in the remaining whites.

Pour into an ungreased 10" springform pan. Bake for 35 minutes, or until a wooden pick inserted in the center comes out clean. Cool on a rack for 45 minutes. Run a knife around the edge to loosen the cake. Remove the cake from the pan and top with the berries.

Microwave the honey on high power for 30 seconds. Stir in the lemon juice and let cool slightly. Drizzle the glaze over the top of the cake and the berries.

PER SERVING: 190 calories, 5 g protein, 39 g carbohydrates, 2 g total fat, 0.5 g saturated fat, 3 g fiber, 82 mg sodium

EASY RED VELVET CAKE

Decorate this cake to suit the occasion. Chocolate curls and strawberry halves are perfect for Mother's Day. Top with jelly beans for Easter or candy corn for Halloween. Candy mint leaves and Red Hots make holly for a lovely Christmas cake.

Makes 16 servings

1 package (18.2 ounces) red velvet cake mix

1 cup light mayonnaise

3 large egg whites

1 cup water

1 container (8 ounces) fat-free or light frozen whipped topping, thawed

Preheat the oven to 350°F. Coat two 8" cake pans with cooking spray. Sprinkle with 1 teaspoon of the cake mix; shake the pans to coat.

Whisk together the remaining cake mix, mayonnaise, egg whites, and water until well blended. Divide the batter between the pans and bake for 30 minutes, or until a wooden pick inserted in the center comes out clean. Cool in the pans for 5 minutes; remove to a rack to cool completely.

Place one cake layer on a plate. Spread the top of the cake with half of the whipped topping. Repeat with the second layer and remaining topping.

PER SERVING: 339 calories, 4 g protein, 49 g carbohydrates, 13 g total fat, 3 g saturated fat, 1 g fiber, 533 mg sodium

APPLE-CHERRY PIE

Makes 8 servings

2½ pounds apples
(see "Fast and Fresh Ideas for
Apples")

½ cup dried cherries

6 tablespoons honey

3 tablespoons all-purpose
flour

1 tablespoon lemon juice

½ teaspoon ground cinnamon

⅛ teaspoon ground nutmeg

2 store-bought refrigerated
unbaked pie crusts

1 egg, beaten

1 tablespoon decorating sugar

Heat the oven to 375°F with the rack in the center position.

Peel and core the apples. Cut into ⅓"-thick wedges and toss into a bowl with the cherries, honey, flour, lemon juice, cinnamon, and nutmeg.

Line a 10" pie plate with one pie crust. Top with the apple mixture.

Roll out the second crust to 13" diameter and cut a 2¼" hole out of the center.

Put on top of the pie and press the edges of the dough together to seal. Brush the top with the egg and sprinkle with the sugar.

Bake until the apples are tender, about 1 hour.

PER SERVING: 379 calories, 4 g protein, 63 g carbohydrates, 15 g total fat, 6 g saturated fat, 4 g fiber, 290 mg sodium

FAST AND FRESH IDEAS FOR APPLES

Apples are one of the few fruits grown in all 50 states, so it's easy for everyone to find locally grown apples. Depending on the variety, taste can range from sweet to tart; try using a mix of types within a recipe for best results. To save money, purchase all-purpose Golden Delicious, Granny Smith, and McIntosh, which are good for both cooking and snacking, and buy in bulk. Apples get high marks for heart health: They supply fiber (including a soluble type called pectin) and antioxidants and may help lower cholesterol naturally.

EASY PUMPKIN PIE

The superquick prep on this pumpkin pie makes it an easy option
any night of the week. Offer whipped topping on the side.

Makes 8 servings

1 cup canned pumpkin puree

3 eggs

1 cup evaporated milk

¾ cup packed brown sugar

½ teaspoon ground cinnamon

½ teaspoon ground ginger

⅛ teaspoon ground nutmeg

⅛ teaspoon ground allspice

1 prepared unbaked pie crust

Preheat the oven to 375°F.

Whisk together the pumpkin, eggs, milk, sugar,
cinnamon, ginger, nutmeg, and allspice in a large
bowl. Pour into the unbaked crust.

Bake for 40 to 45 minutes, or until the center of
the filling is set. Cool before serving.

PER SERVING: 222 calories, 6 g protein, 35 g carbohydrates,
7 g total fat, 2 g saturated fat, 1 g fiber, 172 mg sodium

Alternate: You can turn Easy Pumpkin Pie into Praline Pumpkin Pie. Before filling the
pie crust with the pumpkin mixture, add a layer of praline. To make the praline, cut 2
teaspoons butter into ¼ cup packed brown sugar. Stir in 1 tablespoon maple syrup
and ⅓ cup chopped toasted pecans. Press the praline mixture evenly into the bottom
of the unbaked pie crust. Bake at 425°F for 10 minutes. Remove from the oven, allow
to cool, and then fill with the pumpkin mixture. Bake as directed. Makes
8 servings.

CHOCOLATE RASPBERRY TOWERS
WITH SAUCE

Unlike commercially made fudge sauces, there are no hydrogenated oils in this sauce.

Makes 12 servings

½ cup boiling water

½ cup unsweetened cocoa powder (we used Ghirardelli)

1 cup dark brown sugar

¾ cup reduced-fat sour cream

5 tablespoons unsalted butter, cut into pieces

1 teaspoon vanilla extract

4 tablespoons framboise (raspberry liqueur) or Chambord, divided

2 large eggs

1¼ cups all-purpose flour

1 teaspoon baking soda

Pinch of salt

2–3 cups fresh raspberries

4 ounces bittersweet chocolate, melted

Heat the oven to 350°F. Coat a 9" x 9" baking pan with cooking spray.

Whisk together the boiling water and the cocoa in a large bowl until smooth. Add the sugar, sour cream, butter, vanilla, and 2 tablespoons of the framboise or Chambord and whisk until smooth. Whisk in the eggs one at a time until well incorporated. Whisk the flour, baking soda, and the salt in a small bowl and add to the batter. Whisk until just combined.

Pour into the prepared pan. Bake until the cake is beginning to pull away from the sides of the pan and a wooden pick comes out clean, about 25 minutes. Cool in the pan for 10 minutes. Invert onto a rack and then flip again onto another rack to cool.

Cut the cake into 12 rectangles and split each piece horizontally. Brush the cut sides of the cake with the remaining 2 tablespoons framboise or Chambord. Arrange the bottom slices cut side up on serving plates and top each with 6 to 9 raspberries, standing them upright. Top with the remaining cake halves. Pour the melted chocolate over each tower, letting it drip down the sides, and serve.

PER SERVING: 280 calories, 5 g protein, 39 g carbohydrates, 13 g total fat, 7 g saturated fat, 2 g fiber, 146 mg sodium

CRISPY RICE CHOCOLATE POPS

The slightly chewy texture of these fun pops means you must savor them slowly.

Makes 16 servings

3 tablespoons unsalted butter

1 package (10 ounces) marshmallows

2 teaspoons vanilla extract

6 cups organic puffed brown rice cereal

8 ounces bittersweet chocolate, melted

½ cup finely chopped pistachios

½ cup unsweetened coconut flakes, toasted

Melt the butter in a large pot over medium heat. Add the marshmallows and stir until melted, about 6 minutes. Turn off the heat, stir in the vanilla and cereal until combined. Transfer to a baking sheet coated with cooking spray. Let stand until cool enough to handle, about 5 minutes.

Form the mixture with damp hands into 32 equal balls (about 2" diameter). Stick a small bamboo skewer into each ball, pressing gently to adhere.

Transfer the pops to a large sheet of oiled foil and let them stand for about 15 minutes.

Dip each pop in the melted chocolate and return to the foil. Let them stand for about 10 minutes. Sprinkle half of the pops with the pistachios and the other half with the coconut.

PER SERVING: 232 calories, 3 g protein, 33 g carbohydrates, 12 g total fat, 6 g saturated fat, 2 g fiber, 67 mg sodium

CHOCOLATE CHERRY CUPCAKES WITH VANILLA BEAN FROSTING

Join the cupcake craze! They're a cute, no-deprivation way
to keep portions under control.

Makes 16 cupcakes

1 cup dried cherries

1 cup water

1 cup unsweetened cocoa powder

4 ounces bittersweet chocolate, broken

2 tablespoons unsalted butter

¾ cup light brown sugar

1 teaspoon vanilla extract

Pinch of salt

4 large eggs

½ cup all-purpose flour

1 teaspoon baking soda

2 vanilla beans, split

8 ounces reduced-fat cream cheese (Neufchâtel), at room temperature

½ cup + 1 tablespoon confectioners' sugar

Heat the oven to 350°F. Line 2 muffin pans with 16 paper liners.

Combine the cherries and water in a saucepan. Bring to a boil. Transfer to a food processor. Add the cocoa, chocolate, and butter and pulse until combined. Cool for 1 minute. Add the brown sugar, vanilla, and the salt and puree until almost smooth.

Pulse in the eggs until well combined. Whisk together the flour and baking soda in a bowl and add to the food processor. Pulse until just combined.

Divide the batter evenly among the pans. Bake in the upper and lower thirds of the oven until the tops are slightly domed and firm to the touch, 18 to 20 minutes. Cool the cupcakes in the pans on a rack for 10 minutes. Remove from the pans and cool completely on the rack.

Scrape the vanilla bean seeds into a bowl. Add the cream cheese and confectioners' sugar and beat well. Pipe or spread the frosting onto the cupcakes.

PER SERVING: 219 calories, 5 g protein, 31 g carbohydrates, 10 g total fat, 5 g saturated fat, 4 g fiber, 170 mg sodium

"BAKED" APPLE HALVES WITH MAPLE CREAM

Bake the apples up to a day ahead, cool, and store them in the refrigerator, covered.
Great apples for this dish include Ida Reds, Jonathan, and Jonagold.

Makes 4 servings

2 large apples, halved lengthwise and cored (see note)

4 teaspoons butter or trans-free margarine, cut into small pieces

½ cup orange juice

1 tablespoon apple cider vinegar

¼ cup evaporated milk

2 tablespoons maple syrup

Place a small mixing bowl in the refrigerator until needed.

Place the apples, skin side down, in a 4- to 6-quart slow cooker and dot with the butter. Mix the orange juice and vinegar and pour over the top.

Cover and cook on low for 2 to 3 hours, or until the apples are soft but still hold their shape. Remove to a plate. Pour the juice from the cooker into a small saucepan. Bring to a boil and boil for 3 to 4 minutes, or until the liquid is thick and syrupy. Set aside.

Whip the milk and maple syrup in the chilled bowl with an electric mixer on high speed for 3 to 5 minutes, or until thickened.

Top each apple half with 1½ tablespoons of the maple cream and drizzle with 1 tablespoon of the reserved fruit syrup.

PER SERVING: 154 calories, 2 g protein, 27 g carbohydrates, 5 g total fat, 3 g saturated fat, 3 g fiber, 47 mg sodium

FRUIT FREEZE

Similar to granita, this fat-free fruit dessert is the perfect ending to a spicy meal.

Makes 8 servings

1 can (15 ounces) peaches packed in juice

1 can (6 ounces) pineapple juice

1½ frozen bananas

Place the peaches with juice, pineapple juice, and bananas in a blender or food processor and pulse until well blended. Place the blender or food processor container in the freezer for 4 hours.

Return the container to its base and whip the mixture. If not serving immediately, pour into a freezer container until ready to use.

PER SERVING: 54 calories, 1 g protein, 14 g carbohydrates, 0 g total fat, 0 g saturated fat, 1 g fiber, 3 mg sodium

STAINED-GLASS COOKIES

The tops of these pretty, colorful cookies are not hard to cut out.
Choose a larger round cookie cutter and a smaller heart- or star-shaped cutter.
The round shape is to cut out the "doughnut" and the smaller cutter is to cut
out the doughnut's hole. These are cookies for special occasions, but
worth the time. They are not too sweet and very attractive.

Makes 18 cookies

2 cups all-purpose flour

⅔ cup reduced-calorie trans-free margarine

½ teaspoon almond extract

6 tablespoons unsweetened apple juice or cranberry juice

½ cup jelly or fruit puree (any flavor)

Combine the flour, margarine, and almond extract in a large bowl with a pastry blender or two knives. Add the juice, 1 tablespoon at a time, stirring, until a soft dough forms.

Wrap the dough in plastic wrap and refrigerate until firm, 2 hours or overnight.

Preheat the oven to 350°F.

Roll the dough to a ⅛" thickness. Cut into 2½" rounds with a large round cookie cutter. With a smaller cutter, cut out a heart or star in the center of half of the rounds. Remove each heart or star shape, leaving a hole in the center. Discard the hearts or stars.

Transfer the cookies to baking sheets with a metal spatula and bake for about 10 minutes, or until just slightly golden. Cool the cookies on the sheets for 2 to 3 minutes. Place about ¼ teaspoon jelly in the center of each solid cookie (the jelly will melt slightly with the warmth of the cookie). Top each with a cutout cookie and press gently around the edges so the cookies stick together. Transfer to a wire rack and cool completely. Store the cookies between layers of plastic wrap in a cool place.

PER SERVING: 125 calories, 1 g protein, 17 g carbohydrates, 6 g total fat, 2 g saturated fat, 1 g fiber, 54 mg sodium

Part 3

FITNESS
MOVES

CHAPTER 12

Shoe Solutions

Walk this way: The wrong shoes slow you down, make you fat, and set you up for a lifetime of injuries. Check out our lab, and you'll never shop the same way again.

The shoes you wear can make you feel slim, sexy, and stylish—or they can leave you wincing in pain. Did you ever wonder how much damage you are doing to your feet when you walk to work in sky-high heels or scuff through errands in flip-flops?

We wanted to find out for sure, so we took three 40-something women to a high-tech motion-analysis laboratory to test out four different types of shoes: flip-flops, high heels, dress flats, and toning sneakers. (Results were compared with our gold standard of comfort—a simple pair of running shoes.) At the lab, the women were outfitted with sensors to measure muscle and joint activity so we could see precisely what types of stress their bodies were subjected to. Read on to learn the findings and (because we know shoe choice is not always based purely on practicalities) get expert advice on how to make even those stilettos as foot-healthy and pain free as possible.

FLIP-FLOPS

Flip-Flops Lab Result:

Our testers were up to 2.5 times less stable in flip-flops than sneakers

They may be your favorite things to slip on as soon as the weather gets warm, but flip-flops aren't as foot-friendly as you might think. Here's why:

Scrunch time: Only a thin strap and your bunched toes keep flip-flops from coming off. That constant grip makes it impossible for your arch to flex normally, which in turn compromises the way your forefoot pushes off when you step forward. Deprived of a powerful push-off, our testers compensated by using their hips, forcing their knees and hips to absorb more impact. In addition, your butt and the backs of your legs are less engaged in your stride, weakening those muscles over time, says Katy Bowman, a biomechanical scientist and the author of *Every Woman's Guide to Foot Pain Relief.*

Short steppin': Wearing flip-flops shortens your gait, so you can't expect to get very far very fast in them. Eventually, your shortened stride may lead to lower-body fatigue, which in turn may make you more inclined to hop in a cab or get in your car rather than hoof it, says Philip J. Vasyli, a podiatrist and the founder of the orthotic company Vasyli International in San Rafael, California.

Flip-Flop Fixes

Stretch it out. To help your toes recover from the stress of being clenched, stretch the muscles along the top of the foot, says Bowman. Stand with your feet hip-width apart, then place one foot behind you, turning the tops of your toes to the floor. Try to keep both knees straight, stand tall, and don't let your ankle roll out to the side as you stretch. Start by holding the stretch for a few seconds on each side (your foot might cramp initially because it's not used to stretching this way), and work up to 60 seconds on each side.

Shop smarter. If you can't fathom going through a flip-flop-less summer, opt for a more structured pair. Look for a contoured arch that fits to the shape of your foot (brands to buy: Chaco, Reef, Orthaheel, and Dansko, all of which have the American Podiatric Medical Association's seal of acceptance) rather than the flimsy corner-drugstore ones that look like they're stamped out of a piece of rubber.

THE HEEL DEAL

High Heels Lab Result:
Testers walked slower in heels than sneakers. Wear them daily and the decrease in calorie burn could add up to a 5-pound gain in a year!

There's good reason most women willingly forgo comfort to squeeze their feet into stilettos: Adding inches makes you look slimmer, accentuates calf muscles, and even lifts your backside.

But you may be doing lasting damage if you live your life in heels. A 2011 Danish study found that walking in heels can increase the risk of osteoarthritis sixfold. Here's what else we found in testing.

Tighter quads: Imagine standing on the edge of a ski slope with your toes pointing downhill. To compensate for this tipped-forward position, it's natural to bend your knees slightly and arch your back. As a result, your quads are forced to work overtime, which makes them tight and prone to injury. Walking with your knees slightly bent also puts 200 percent more stress on your kneecaps, which can wear away at the cartilage and increase your risk of developing arthritis, says Howard Dananberg, DPM, a podiatrist in Bedford, New Hampshire.

Screaming shins: The added height of heels puts extra strain on the shin muscles, which control the forefoot. This repetitive strain can eventually lead to painful shin splints.

Knotty calves: Heels put your calf muscles in a shortened position. Over time, this can become permanent: One study in the *Journal of Experimental Biology* found regular heel wearers had calf muscles that were an average of 13 percent shorter than those of nonheel wearers, making it uncomfortable for them to walk without heels because their natural stride was thrown off.

17

THE NUMBER OF PAIRS OF SHOES THE AVERAGE AMERICAN WOMAN OWNS

Heels Help

Stretch it out. Give your calves a good daily stretch like this one from Bowman: Stand with your feet hip-width apart and place a rolled-up towel under the ball of your right foot. Lower your right heel to the floor. Once you're comfortable here, take a small step forward with your left foot, keeping your hips square. Hold for 20 to 30 seconds and work up to 60 seconds.

Massage your shins. Relieve shin pain with a gentle self-rubdown, applying long vertical finger strokes down the front of your lower leg. Then focus on kneading the muscles horizontally, says Bowman.

Embrace the commuter shoe. Switch to low-heeled options for getting places, and save those skyscrapers for when you're mostly sitting pretty.

Shop smarter. Feet swell over the day, so if a shoe feels slightly tight at 7:00 a.m., it'll be a vise by nightfall. Only buy shoes that are roomy enough, and consider going lower. Research shows that 2-inch heels create impact forces 4 percent greater than flats, while 3-inch heels boost stress by 33 percent.

FLAT ATTACK

Flats Lab Result:

In our tests, women put about 25 percent more impact on the heel with each step when wearing flats, compared with pumps.

Flats sound like the healthier alternative to heels, but the truth is that even a basic ballet flat or canvas casual can be just as problematic, says Megan Leahy, DPM, a podiatrist with the Illinois Bone & Joint Institute in Chicago.

Arch enemy: Many flats lack internal support (like the kind you find in a sneaker). Without it, the ligaments and tendons along the bottom of your foot can overstretch and the arch can collapse, says Marlene Reid, DPM, a podiatric surgeon in Naperville, Illinois. This in turn can lead to the painful foot condition plantar fasciitis—a notoriously hard-to-treat burning or aching along the bottom of the foot. Poor internal support is especially problematic if you're naturally flat-footed.

Strained soles: Many casual flats have even less interior cushioning than heels or sandals. This lack of padding can trigger pain in the heel or ball of your foot when you're walking, especially if you have high arches, says Dr. Leahy.

Flat Fixes

Give your feet a workout. To wear shoes with no built-in support, you need to strengthen the tiny foot muscles that support your arches, says Bowman. Try doing toe lifts: Raise your big toe without moving the rest of the gang. It might seem impossible at first, but it's like riding a bike, says Bowman: You just have to master the coordination. Until you get the knack, wiggle your toes and rub your feet vigorously, which will stimulate your nerve endings and help wake up your feet. Do 20 toe lifts per foot.

Stretch it out. Just as the abductor/adductor machine at the gym strengthens your outer and inner thighs, you can work your toe abductors and adductors to make the muscles of your foot stronger and more supportive. Start by interlacing your fingers with your toes to help press them apart, then spread and relax them without assistance from your hands. Hold the stretch long enough to sing the alphabet. Do this once a day (or up to three times if you have bunions).

Bump it up. Help strengthen the small muscles in your feet and lower legs by striding barefoot across an uneven surface such as cobblestones. This also helps stimulate the nerves in your feet. Buy a pre-made cobblestone mat with smooth stones already glued to it ($60, amazon.com), or find (or make) a bumpy space to walk back and forth on in your backyard.

Add OTC insoles. If you have flat feet (your wet footprint shows the entire foot), foam or rubber insoles can help prevent your arches from collapsing. If you have high arches (you see only the heel and ball of your foot in your foot-print), look for an insole with more rigid arch support.

Shop smarter. Look for flats with an insole that curves along the same lines as your foot and arch. Then try to fold the shoe in half—it should bend only at the ball (the same place your foot naturally bends as you walk). Also avoid pairs that fold right in the middle or roll up easily.

ROCKER SHOCKER

Rockers Lab Result:

Surprise! Our testers worked their butt and thigh muscles less when wearing tone-up shoes, compared with simple sneakers.

Shoes with rounded or "rocker" soles that purportedly increase muscle activity and boost calorie burn are big business. After all, who doesn't want to get a workout without really working out? But despite their medical provenance (rocker-bottom shoes were originally engineered to help patients with pain in the balls of the feet, says Dr. Leahy), consider the following before you get a pair as a fitness tool.

Stress case: The rigid soles prevent arches from naturally flexing. Eventually, this can cause your arches to flatten and lead to overpronation (when the feet excessively roll in while walking). The result: Your feet absorb less shock, causing your knees and back to take on extra stress.

Teeter trouble: Testers were slightly less stable in the rocker-bottom shoes. The Consumer Product Safety Commission's Web site is loaded with complaints about injuries from toning shoes (including tendinitis; foot, leg, and hip pain; and even broken bones resulting from falls). And Reebok recently agreed to hand over $25 million in consumer refunds for overstating the benefits of its toning shoes.

Rocker Relief

Be inspired (but don't skip your strength workout). If these shoes help you feel more conscious of the benefits of every step you take and make you want to walk more, go for it! But don't skip proven strengtheners. The best way to tone

43

THE PERCENTAGE OF WOMEN WHO SAY THEY HAVE SUFFERED SHOE INJURIES

your lower body is with strength moves such as squats and lunges, not just walking around in toning shoes.

Work your wobble muscles. Because these shoes make you unstable, they can lead to ankle injury. To strengthen the muscles around the ankle, practice standing barefoot with one leg lifted, keeping your standing knee straight, and try to minimize wobbling. Start with 30 seconds and work up to 60 seconds at a time.

Take it slow. The convex soles force you to change your natural gait, so it can take your muscles a while to get used to the movement. "At first you should not wear these shoes all day, every day," says Dr. Leahy. Start with about an hour a day and build up gradually. And listen to your body: "If you start to develop pain in your back, hips, knees, feet, or ankles, switch shoes," she adds.

Shop smarter. If you're determined to try the rocker technology, look for a pair that actually bends at the ball of the foot. This will allow your foot to flex more naturally despite the extra thickness of the sole.

IS IT TIME FOR NEW SHOES?

Athletic walking shoes should be replaced after they've logged 350 to 600 miles. If you walk 3 miles 5 days a week, that means every 6 to 10 months. To keep track, write the date you started using a pair in marker on the inside of the shoe's tongue.

PUT YOUR BEST FOOT FORWARD

Bulky, stiff sneakers are out, and comfort is in! The latest research shows that athletic shoes that overrestrict foot motion may contribute to injuries, and so can flimsy flats. We asked 33 walkers to test more than 100 pairs for the right balance of support and flexibility for any occasion to come up with this top list. To keep your feet feeling good mile after mile, try a bunch on and go with the shoe that feels best on your feet. Here are our top picks.

Athletic Shoes

Lace up one of these top picks for working out.

BEST FOR HIKING: Ahnu Rockridge II ($110, also available in green, brown; ahnu.com) These lightweight hikers perform as well as bulkier high-top versions. "They're much more flexible," reports tester Jess Lee, 30, of Brooklyn. The rugged sole grips as you go up and down hills but is bendable enough that you can keep up a smooth, rolling stride on level terrain. And the reinforced toe area protects your feet from bumps against rocks and roots.

BEST FOR FAST WALKING: New Balance 860 ($90, also available in blue; shopnewbalance.com) This shoe has a superflexible toe that makes it easy to push off and quicken your pace. But no matter how fast you go, the ankle padding will keep your heel snugly in place. "My foot didn't budge, even in thin socks," reports tester Jessica Branch, 45, of New York City. A mesh upper is lined to buffer cold and wind.

BEST FOR BUNIONS: Asics Gel-Tech Walker Neo 2 ($100; asicsamerica.com) An ultraroomy toe box and an expandable "bunion window" on the inside take the squeeze off swollen joints and toes. "I could walk longer than usual, because the shoe has a lot of give in the right place," says bunion sufferer Connie Esmond, 63, of Broken Arrow, Oklahoma.

BEST FOR OVERWEIGHT WALKERS: Reebok DMX Max ReeDirect ($70, also available in white; reebok.com) Air pockets in the rubber bottom of the shoe reduce impact for more comfort and less chance of injury. Even slim walkers enjoy the extra cushioning, especially for long walks. "No matter how far I went, my feet never got sore," reports tester Jennifer DeLuca, 41, of Brooklyn. The mesh upper lets air circulate so feet stay dry and cool.

BEST FOR RUNNING INTERVALS: Brooks Trance 11 ($140; brooksrunning.com) Walkers who want to add jogging bursts should opt for a running shoe. This one is designed for high impact but is still flexible enough for the rolling motion of walking. "These shoes were comfortable at any speed; I felt like they really sprang me forward," reports tester Molly Raisch, 23, of Allentown, Pennsylvania.

Casual Shoes

Slip on these shoes for more everyday wear.

BEST FOR RUNNING ERRANDS: Saucony Bullet ($60, available in 10 colors; saucony.com) These stylish sneakers are lightweight and have just enough arch support to keep your feet comfy when you're on the go. "I wore these for shopping and doing errands—they were just right for every day," reports tester Eileen Kohn, 48, of Aurora, Ohio. The full coverage makes them a good choice for spring and fall.

BEST FOR DRESSING UP: Hush Puppies Veracity ($85; hushpuppies.com) These shoes have a hip look, thanks to the asymmetrical strap, yet they provide the comfort of sneakers with cushioned insoles and arch support. "I could walk for longer than I can in flats," says Jodi Standish, 32, of Bellevue, Nebraska. "My heels and arches felt great." The leather upper molds to your foot after a few wears for a snug—but not tight—fit.

BEST FOR ALL-DAY WEAR: Scarpa Caipirinha ($130, also available in pink, tan; scarpa.com) These casual sneakers are sturdier than they look, making them a comfy choice for activities such as sightseeing, when you're on your feet for hours. The sole—made of slip-resistant Vibram rubber—is firm in the back and flexible in the front. "I usually take off my shoes as soon as I get home, but I wore these late into the night without even noticing," says Kristina Donatelli, 39, of Bethlehem, Pennsylvania.

CHAPTER 13

Raising the Barre

Get lean and sculpted—and drop up to 3½ pounds a week!—with our 25-day Ballet Boot Camp Challenge.

You don't have to be able to arabesque in pointe shoes to get the graceful, sculpted body of a dancer. What you do need: our fat-blasting Ballet Boot Camp Challenge. Created by Sadie Lincoln, founder of Barre3 exercise studios, these moves combine yoga, Pilates, light weights, and a secret weapon that in-the-know exercisers (including celebs like Ricki Lake) swear by—barre work. You don't even have to leave home to get the body-slimming benefits: The ballet-derived exercises are normally done using a stationary handrail, but you can do them with a chair or kitchen table.

What makes this workout so effective? It strengthens your deepest belly muscles, pulling in your waist like a corset, while lifting your butt, trimming your thighs, and toning your arms. It also whips into shape your perfect-posture muscles, so you'll stand straighter after a single session.

We know it works because we tested the plan on real women. For 25 days, they followed our Ballet Boot Camp Challenge, as well as eating guidelines and recipes recommended by Andrea Nakayama, a nutritionist in Portland, Oregon (find them at prevention.com/barre-workout-recipes). The final results were

181

astonishing: One woman lost 9 pounds in 13 days, another trimmed her hips by more than 2 inches and whittled her waist by 3 inches, and testers' upper arms shrank by up to 1 ½ inches! The group also saw improvements in grace and balance and even had less lower-back pain.

YOUR BALLET BOOT CAMP CHALLENGE

Aim to do the Ballet Boot Camp moves 3 or 4 times a week and Your-Choice Cardio sessions 2 or 3 times each week. Feel free to swap days according to your schedule.

DAY 1	DAY 2	DAY 3	DAY 4	DAY 5	DAY 6	DAY 7
Ballet Boot Camp	Ballet Boot Camp and Your-Choice Cardio	Your-Choice Cardio	Ballet Boot Camp	Your Choice Cardio	Ballet Boot Camp	Rest

YOUR-CHOICE CARDIO

To speed your slim-down, include at least 30 minutes of moderate- to high-intensity cardio 2 or 3 times per week. Boost your burn by incorporating intervals: Alternate bursts of faster walking (or whatever aerobic exercise you like best) with bouts at a slower pace. Here's a calorie-torching interval workout to get you started.

WARMUP	INTERVALS	COOLDOWN
3 MINUTES	25 MINUTES	2 MINUTES
3 to 4 (effort level*)	Alternate between 1 minute at 7 to 8 and 1 minute at 5 to 6	3 to 4

Note: Gauge your effort on a scale of 1 to 10: "10" is working as hard as you can; "1" is sitting on the couch.

GEAR YOU NEED AND HOW TO USE IT

- A barre or another waist-level surface. Your kitchen counter or the back of a sturdy chair are great options.
- A 9-inch exercise ball
- 1- to 3-pound dumbbells

Warm up by marching in place for 2 to 3 minutes. Then perform 1 set of each move, unless otherwise noted. (Too many reps? Start gradually and work your way up, or try the moves without weights.) For best results, do the moves slowly and with control: Perfect form, not speed, will help you slip into your skinny jeans faster! Cool down with 5 minutes of full-body stretching.

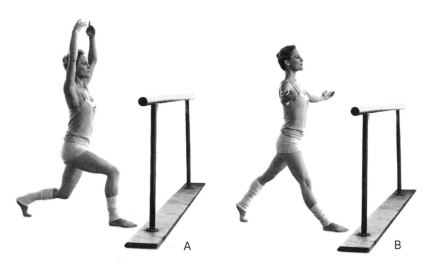

A   B

CAROUSEL HORSE
TARGETS THIGHS, BUTT, ARMS, BACK

Stand facing the barre, with your feet parallel and hip-distance apart. Step back with your left leg, bending your right knee about 90 degrees and keeping it over your ankle, and lift your arms overhead. Pressing your feet into the floor, bend your left knee toward the floor and lower your hips a few inches. This is your starting position (A). Open your arms out to the sides while straightening your legs, keeping your left heel lifted (B). Return to the starting position. Do 30 reps. Switch legs and repeat.

Make it easier: Rest your hands lightly on the barre throughout the move.

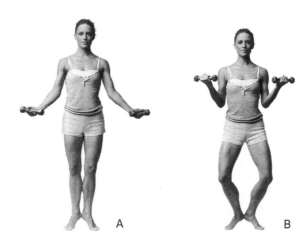

A   B

ATHLETIC FIRST-POSITION BICEPS CURL
TARGETS THIGHS, CORE, FRONT OF ARMS

Holding dumbbells with your palms up, stand with your heels together and your toes
pointing out slightly. Lift your heels about 1 inch off of the floor and press them
together. This is your starting position (A). Bend your knees slightly as you curl the
weights toward your shoulders (B). Return to the starting position. Do 30 reps.

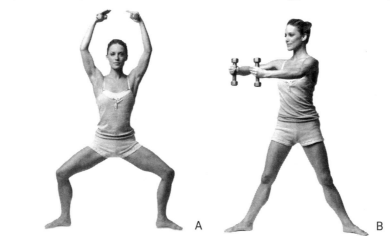

A   B

DANCER'S TWIST
TARGETS THIGHS, WAIST, SHOULDERS, BACK

Holding the weights, stand with your feet wider than shoulder-distance apart and
your toes turned out slightly. Bend your knees about 90 degrees and lift your arms
overhead. This is your starting position (A). Straighten your legs to stand, slowly
twisting to the right as you lower your arms to chest height (B). Return to the starting
position and repeat the twist on the opposite side. That's 1 rep. Do 20 reps.

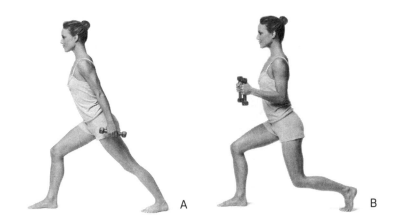

A   B

TRICEPS LIFTS IN CRESCENT LUNGE
TARGETS LEGS, BUTT, ARMS, BACK

Holding dumbbells with your arms at your sides, step your left foot back, bending your right knee and hinging your torso forward (A). Bend your elbows about 90 degrees, lowering your left knee toward the floor (B). Return to the starting position, squeezing your triceps to straighten your arms. Do 30 reps. Switch legs and repeat.

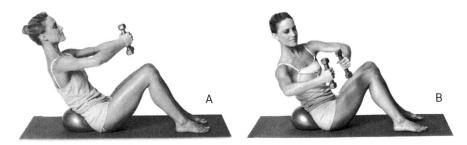

A   B

OBLIQUE TWIST
TARGETS WAIST, CORE, SHOULDERS, BACK

Sit on the floor with your knees bent, your feet flat, and the ball behind your lower back. Holding the dumbbells, with your elbows bent slightly, lean back into the ball (A). Slowly twist to the right (B). Rotate to the center and then twist to the left. That's 1 rep. Do 20 reps.

 I DID IT!

"My stomach is flat for the first time in my life!"

—Misty Tomples, 38, who lost 3½ inches off her waist in 25 days

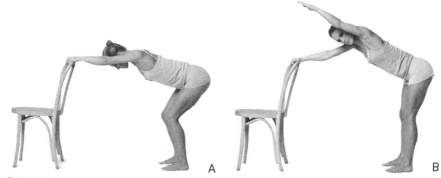

SWIM
TARGETS CORE, BACK

Place your palms shoulder-width apart on the barre and bend forward. Keeping your back straight, walk your feet back until they're under your hips, with your knees slightly bent (A). Engage your core and press your palms into the barre. Straighten your legs, lifting your left arm and rotating your chest to the left (B). Repeat on the opposite side. Alternate arms for 1 minute. Do 2 sets.

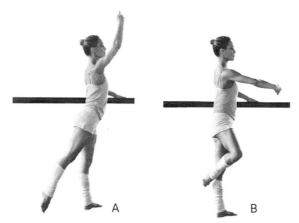

BALLET LEG LIFT
TARGETS THIGHS, BUTT, CORE, BACK

Stand with your heels together, your toes 3 to 4 inches apart, and your left hand resting lightly on the barre. Extend your right leg back with your toes pointed while raising your right arm, with your elbow slightly bent. Keep your hips facing forward, your pelvis tucked under, and your abs drawn in. This is your starting position (A). Draw your right foot toward your left calf, engaging your core, and lower your right arm to chest height (B). Return to the starting position. Do 20 reps. Repeat on the opposite side.

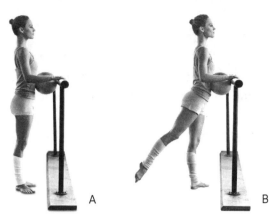

A   B

STANDING SEAT WORK
TARGETS BUTT, THIGHS, CORE

Stand facing the barre, with your heels together and your toes 3 to 4 inches apart. Place the ball between your belly and the barre and draw your navel toward your spine (A). Step back with your right foot, with your heel lifted and the top of your big toe on the floor. Engage your abs and raise your right leg a few inches, lifting from your glutes (B). Lower your right leg 1 inch and lift again. Do a total of 60 pulses. Switch legs and repeat.

Get more out of your move! On your final rep, keep your back leg lifted and hold for 15 to 30 seconds.

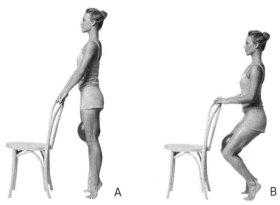

A   B

POWER LEG PULSE
TARGETS THIGHS, CALVES

Stand with your feet parallel and hip-distance apart, with the ball between your inner thighs and your hands resting lightly on the barre. Squeeze the ball with your thighs and lift your heels (A). Bend your knees. Holding here, pulse down and up about 1 inch, keeping your heels lifted throughout (B). Do 50 reps.

Get more out of your move! Finish by holding the lowered position for 30 seconds.

*"I now walk with grace and confidence,
and I'm wearing clothes that have been
in the closet for 10 years!"*

—Susie Desmond, 68, who lost almost 13 pounds in 25 days

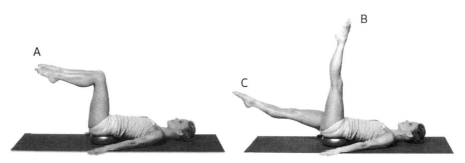

SCISSORS
TARGETS CORE

Lie on your back with your knees bent, the ball under your hips, and your arms out to the sides. Lift your feet so your shins are parallel with the floor, with your knees stacked over your hips (A), and then extend your legs straight up (B). This is your starting position. Lower your right leg, keeping your toes pointed (C). Return to the starting position, and then lower and lift your left leg. That's 1 rep. Do 25 reps.

BUT WAIT, THERE'S MORE

You can watch a video of this workout at prevention.com/barre-workout-video.

GET A LEG UP!

While you're toning your legs with our Ballet Boot Camp Challenge, use these tips to make them soft, smooth, and cellulite free! Whether the issue is unwanted hair, cellulite, or visible veins, this guide will help your legs look great.

Fight Fuzz

Hair growth on your legs typically slows with age, but the bad news? Because the skin on your legs also gets drier, fuzz removal is more likely to cause irritation.

Fast fix: Razors are the gold standard for quick, easy hair removal. "Pick one with multiple blades to get the job done in fewer strokes and minimize nicks and razor burn," says Arielle Kauvar, MD, clinical professor of dermatology at New York University Langone Medical Center in New York City. Try Schick Intuition Naturals Sensitive Care ($9.50; drugstores), with four blades centered in a skin-conditioning solid that melts onto wet skin as you shave.

Firm Up

Got cellulite? You're not alone; more than 85 percent of women experience dimpling, which gets worse with age—perhaps because skin's connective tissue weakens, allowing underlying fat to bulge.

Fast fix: A lotion with theophylline (a diuretic agent) or caffeine—such as Vichy CelluDestock ($39.50; drugstores)—can temporarily plump skin's surface, so legs appear smoother. And a tinted leg spray, like MAC Skinsheen Leg Spray ($28; maccosmetics.com), disguises the lumpy texture but is easier to use than self-tanner because it washes off at the end of the day. Another temporary fix: Do an inverted yoga pose (prevention.com/inverted for how-to's); it can drain excess fluid from fat cells, improving puckering for a few hours.

Vanquish Veins

About 50 percent of women 50-plus have spider veins, small, dilated blood vessels that are visible when located near your skin's surface. The usual cause is genetics, but obesity and long hours of standing or sitting with legs crossed can also cause them by compromising blood flow.

Fast fix: Hide veins with a tinted leg spray or waterproof body makeup, like Dermablend Leg and Body Cover SPF 15 ($27; dermablend.com).

CHAPTER 14

Twice the Workout in Half the Time

No more excuses! Here are five fast workouts to blast fat and firm your trouble spots. You'll get 30 minutes of burn in 15 minutes or less.

In less time than it takes to answer a few e-mails or make a cup of tea, you could burn as many calories as you would going for a brisk 1 ½-mile walk. The key is to up your intensity with more speed or incline and work lots of muscles simultaneously. The following power-packed routines deliver short but sweaty workouts that nudge you out of your comfort zone just long enough to get results—including toned arms, abs, butt, thighs, and calves.

JUMP ROPE: CALORIE BUSTER

The payoff: You'll burn 113 calories in 10 minutes (about 100 jumps per minute).

What you'll need: A basic rubber or cotton jump rope (about $10 at Target or Amazon.com)

The gist: This childhood favorite builds strong bones and tones your arms, shoulders, and legs. For knee-friendly landings, wear socks and sneakers with good cushioning in the forefoot, and avoid hard surfaces like tile floors. Instead, favor those with some give, such as wood.

To get going: March in place, lifting your knees high for 1 minute to warm up. Then aim to jump at least 5 times in a row. Add on more jumps in sets of 5 until you're jumping for 9 minutes straight.

STAIRCLIMBING: SLIM AND SCULPT

The payoff: You'll burn 114 calories in 10 minutes.

What you'll need: A flight of stairs (12 to 16 steps are ideal) and a watch with a timer or second hand

The gist: Turn any staircase into a body-slimming butt-and-thigh sculptor with this routine from Kathy Alcoba, a personal trainer at Chelsea Piers Sports Center in New York City. Doing this daily will decrease your risk of death from heart disease by 62 percent.

To get going: Do each drill for 1 minute unless otherwise noted.

1. Walk up and down stairs for 2 minutes.
2. Walk up 2 steps at a time. As you step up with one foot, kick your other leg back, squeezing your glutes. Walk down.
3. Run up; walk down.
4. Step up sideways. Facing the right, place your left foot on the first step, raise your right leg out to the side, and lower to the step. Walk down.
5. Repeat #4, facing to the left.
6. Run up 2 steps at a time. Walk down.
7. Do single-leg heel lifts. Stand with only the front of your left foot on the step, with your heel and your right leg hanging off. (Hold a railing lightly if needed for balance.) Press your weight into the ball of your foot and raise your heel, coming up onto your toes. Slowly lower. Do 10 times. Move up 2 steps and repeat with your right leg. Continue alternating legs.
8. Run up, walk down.
9. Walk up and down.

EXCUSE ERASERS

What's that? It's too hot to exercise? Too cold? Too boring? Whatever your excuse, we have some great exercise DVDs to try.

Think of an at-home DVD as your exercise insurance: Even when it's too cold to walk outside or too snowy to drive to the gym, you can get a great workout from the comfort of your own living room. Here fitness coach Chris Freytag shares her favorite picks.

Firm Up Fast

Jackie Warner's Personal Training with Jackie Xtreme Timesaver Training features four short strength-training routines that focus on two body parts at once—such as your thighs and arms. Do them individually or combine all of them for a heart-pumping 30-minute workout.

CHRIS SAYS: Jackie's coaching really helps with at-home form. You'll feel like you have a personal trainer. ($15; amazon.com)

Take a Hike

Pop in a Virtual Active DVD and run past Niagara Falls or hike the Grand Canyon right from your treadmill. An optional on-screen coach tells you when to crank up your pace or incline.

CHRIS SAYS: The scenery is so gorgeous, you'll want to extend your workout. ($20; vafitness.com)

Dance Off Calories

The two 20-minute dance workouts in Hemalayaa Bollywood Party Workout feature moves you might do at an Indian wedding or a nightclub. Not familiar with the style? Think hip circles, lassoing overhead, rolling your shoulders.

CHRIS SAYS: If you like aerobics or dance DVDs, this is a fun change, and it'll really raise your heart rate. ($17; acacialifestyle.com)

TREADMILL FAT BURNER

The payoff: You'll burn up to 180 calories in 15 minutes.

What you'll need: A treadmill

The gist: You can burn up to 5 times more fat by alternating your pace during your workout, compared with just chugging along at the same speed. This high-energy routine from New York–based trainer Brett Hoebel really cranks it by increasing the treadmill's incline as you do 30- and 60-second fast and slow intervals, working your legs and butt along with your heart and lungs.

To get going: Follow this simple program.

TIME	ACTIVITY	SPEED (MPH)	INCLINE
0:00	Moderate walk	3.5	1.0
1:00	Brisk walk or jog	4.0 to 5.0	2.5
2:00	Jog or sprint	5.0 to 7.5	2.5
2:30	Walk or jog	3.5 to 6.0	2.5
3:30	Jog or sprint	5.0 to 7.5	3.0
4:00	Walk or jog	3.5 to 6.0	3.0
5:00	Jog or sprint	5.0 to 7.5	3.5
5:30	Walk or jog	3.5 to 6.0	3.5
6:30	Jog or sprint	5.0 to 7.5	4.0
7:00	Walk or jog	3.5 to 6.0	4.0
8:00	Jog or sprint	5.0 to 7.5	4.5
8:30	Walk or jog	3.5 to 6.0	4.5
9:30	Jog or sprint	5.0 to 7.5	5.0
10:00	Walk or jog	3.5 to 6.0	5.0
11:00	Jog or sprint	5.0 to 7.5	5.5
11:30	Walk or jog	3.5 to 6.0	5.5
12:30	Brisk walk	4.0	3.0
14:00	Moderate walk	3.5	2.0
15:00	Finish		

NO-EQUIPMENT TOTAL-BODY TONER

The payoff: You'll burn 138 calories in 15 minutes.

What you'll need: A watch with a timer or second hand

The gist: Get a cardio workout while you firm your trouble zones with this circuit routine from New York City–based trainer Nikki Glor. Research shows that circuits are great for losing fat and toning muscle in minimal time.

To get going: Jog or march in place, circling your arms overhead and down, for 30 seconds to warm up. Do the exercises below in order, followed by 1 minute of jogging or marching in place—that's 1 circuit. Do 3 circuits total.

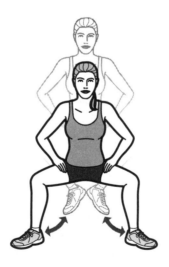

PLIE POP-UP
WORKS INNER THIGHS, QUADS

With your feet wider than shoulder-width apart and your toes pointing out, bend your knees and lower yourself so that your thighs are about parallel with the floor. Pulse 3 times, going up and down just a few inches. On the third pulse, jump and bring your heels together while in the air. Bend your knees into a plie squat again as you land. Repeat for 1 minute.

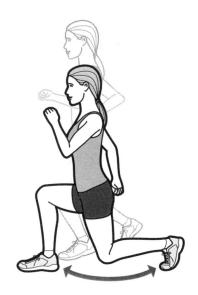

HOP TO JUMPING LUNGE
WORKS QUADS, BUTT

Stand with your right foot about 2 feet in front of your left foot. Jump up and switch
legs. Swing your arms in opposition to your legs. Repeat for 45 seconds. Then do
jumping lunges (shown here) for 15 seconds: Each time you land, bend your knees
90 degrees to lower into a lunge with your front knee over your ankle. Use your arms
to help power you through the jumps.

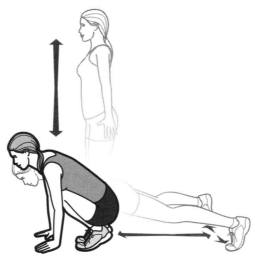

SQUAT THRUST
WORKS LEGS, ARMS, CHEST, ABS

Do 1 jumping jack. Crouch down, placing your hands on the floor. Jump (or walk) your feet back into a plank position (with your feet together, your hands under your shoulders, and your body in line from your head to your heels, with your abs tight). Spring your feet apart, then back together. Jump (or walk) your feet up to your hands and stand up. Repeat for 1 minute.

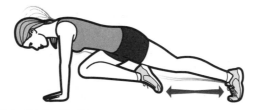

MOUNTAIN CLIMBER
WORKS ARMS, CHEST, ABS

Place your hands on the floor and walk your legs back into a plank position. Quickly pull your right knee into your chest, keeping your spine in line, your hips low, and your abs tight. Switch legs. Alternate legs for 1 minute.

KICKBOXING CARDIO BOOSTER

The payoff: You'll burn 113 calories in 10 minutes.

What you'll need: A watch with a timer or second hand

The gist: Burn stress and fat with this high-energy routine from trainer Jessica Smith, star of the DVD *The 10 Minute Solution: Knockout Body*. You'll fry as many calories as you would running a mile—without the impact—and tone your arms, shoulders, and abs along with your lower body.

To get going:

To warm up, repeat the following for 1 minute:

10 small arm circles forward and back

10 small squats, knees bent, weight over heels

10 front punches, alternating arms

10 knee lifts, alternating legs

Small jumps: For 1 minute, lightly land on balls of feet, shifting weight from foot to foot, arms at sides.

Punch combo: For 1 minute, begin in boxer's stance: fists by chin, elbows pointing down, abs tight, right foot in front. Punch right arm forward. Then

WORK IN A WALK

If you can't hit the pavement as often as you'd like, here's how to sneak in more steps—and slim down faster.

SWEAR OFF SHORTCUTS. Take the long way to your office bathroom or the mall entrance.

RUN ERRANDS—LITERALLY. If you live within a mile of a destination, lace up your shoes and hoof it. You can check distances to restaurants, stores, and more around your home or office at walkscore.com.

STROLL YOUR KIDS OR GRANDKIDS TO SCHOOL. You'll boost everyone's step count and gain quality time together.

SKIP THE ELEVATOR. Stairs burn more calories—and they're often quicker!

turn to left, pivoting on left foot. Punch across body to left. Do twice. Jump to face opposite direction, left foot in front. Repeat with left arm.

Kicks, for 1 minute: In boxer's stance, lift right knee and kick forward, powering it with hips and pushing out through ball of flexed foot. Bend knee as you lower leg. Shift weight to right foot, look over left shoulder, and kick left leg back, keeping knee facing floor, foot flexed, and pushing out through heel. Alternate front and back kicks for 30 seconds. Switch legs and repeat, kicking left leg front and right one back.

Squats, for 1 minute: Stand with feet hip-distance apart. Bend at hips and knees and sit back. Keep knees behind toes. Stand up.

Repeat from small jumps and finish with 1 minute of jumping jacks.

CHAPTER 15

Targeted Toning

Want to blast off back fat, bra rolls, muffin tops, and more? These targeted 5-minute workouts will have you sleek and toned in just 2 weeks.

Technically speaking, your clothes fit. You can zip your jeans (with a little oomph), hook your bra (okay, it stretches), and button your blouses (does anyone really see that little tug?). But you know your wardrobe is on the edge—and not in a good way. Bulges at your armpits, over your waistband, or around your bra band are notorious outfit wreckers. We call them spillover spots, and most of us have them—even otherwise slim women.

But now you can eliminate them: Our targeted workouts laser in on tiny muscles beneath spillover spots that standard moves miss. When eight women tried the plan, they lost an average of 3 pounds and nearly 2 inches off their trouble spots in just 2 weeks. Now it's your turn. You can drop up to 6 pounds in 14 days and look smoother and more streamlined in everything you wear.

SPILLOVER SPOT WORKOUTS

Pick your trouble zone (it may be more than one) and do the prescribed toning moves (see pages 203 to 209) 3 times a week on alternating days to firm up that area.

Combine that with 30 minutes of cardio (see page 208) 5 or 6 times a week to shed fat. (You can do toning and cardio on the same day.)

What you need: A resistance band, mat, and maybe a pair of 3- to 5-pound dumbbells (depending on the routines you choose)

Chris Freytag, certified personal trainer, designed this workout and models the moves.

INSTANT SMOOTHING

While you wait for the toning moves to pay off, keep spillover spots in check with these clever clothing solutions.

GET A PROFESSIONAL BRA FITTING. Experts say 80 percent of women wear the wrong bra size. To prevent your bra from riding up and causing bulges, "choose a bra with a wider band and straps, made out of a supportive but stretchy material," says New York City–based celebrity stylist Katy Robbins.

WEAR A BASE LAYER. Robbins swears by Spanx Slim Cognito Body Shaping Cami made from light compression fabric for smooth, flattering lines. ($74; spanx.com)

TAKE THREE SIZES INTO THE DRESSING ROOM. Wearing clothes that are too tight causes more spillover. To find the most flattering fit, try on the size you think you are, one above it, and one below it, says Marie Denee, founder and editor of *The Curvy Fashionista*.

DON'T BE CLINGY. Thin, body-hugging materials like rayon, light knits, or lightweight cashmere accentuate bulges, while midweight cotton, thick knits, and two-ply fabrics minimize lumps, says Robbins.

FIND YOUR NATURAL WAIST. Stand up straight and bend to the side. The spot at which you bend is your natural waist. For the most flattering look, pants should sit at or just below this point. "The wrong rise [where high pants hit on your waist] quickly kills your look," Denee says.

Firm your upper and middle back to eliminate bra bulges.

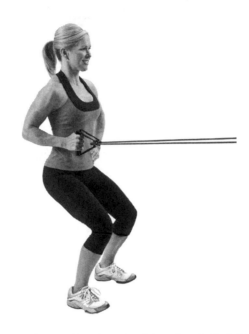

PULSE ROW

Loop a resistance band around a sturdy pole or banister at waist height. Hold both ends in your right hand so that the band is taut and your arm is extended, with your left hand on your hip. Sit back slightly. Squeeze your shoulder blades, bend your elbow, and pull your hand back toward your ribs. Keep your elbow close to your body. Do 10 reps, then hold by your ribs and pulse for 10 reps, releasing and pulling the band only a few inches each time. Repeat with your left arm.

"I lost fat in my chest and back! My bra doesn't feel so tight."

—Colleen Berto, 37; lost 3¼ pounds and 2 inches around her chest and back

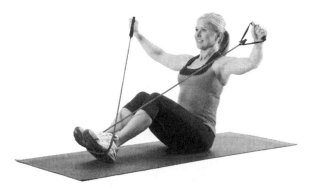

READ THE PAPER

Sit tall with your legs bent and the resistance band wrapped around your feet and crossed in an X. Hold an end in each hand, with your arms out in front of you. Squeeze your shoulder blades together and open your arms to the sides, as if you were opening a newspaper. Keep your abs tight. Slowly return to the starting position. Do 12 to 15 reps.

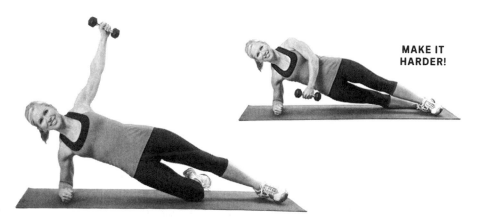

MAKE IT HARDER!

SIDE PLANK WITH ARM SWEEP

Lie on your right side, with your right leg bent, and your left one extended. Prop yourself up on your right elbow. Hold a dumbbell in your left hand with your arm extended in front of you, and the weight near (but not touching) the floor. Squeeze your shoulder blades and raise the dumbbell in an arc toward the ceiling. Slowly lower your arm while holding the plank for all reps. Do 12 to 15 reps on each side.

Make it harder: Extend both of your legs, with your ankles crossed so that your left foot is in front of your right.

Whittle your waist and better define your abs to fit into your jeans again.

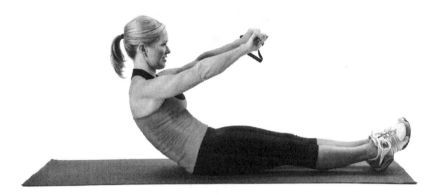

BELLY BUTTON ROLL-UP

Hold the band taut between your hands and lie faceup with your legs extended and your arms overhead. Pull your abs in, lift your arms toward the ceiling, tuck in your chin, and roll your head, shoulders, and torso up and over your legs as far as comfortably possible. Keep your heels firmly on the floor and reach your hands toward your feet. Pause, then slowly roll down onto the floor. Do 5 to 8 reps.

I DID IT!

"My pants are loser and I have more energy."
—Claire Olson, 52; lost 6 pounds and 2½ inches off her waist

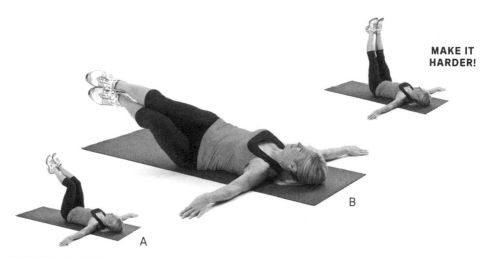

MAKE IT HARDER!

WINDSHIELD WIPER

Lie faceup with your arms out to the sides, with your palms down, and your legs bent 90 degrees so that your feet are off of the floor. Keep your abs tight (A). Slowly lower your legs to the left as far as comfortably possible, keeping your shoulders on the floor (B). Pause, then return to the starting position. Repeat to the right. Do 20 reps, alternating sides.

Make it harder: Do the move with both of your legs extended.

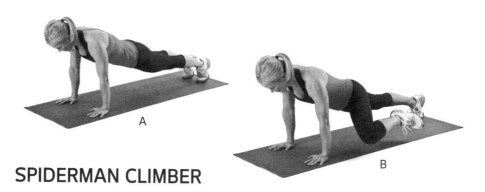

SPIDERMAN CLIMBER

Balance in the plank position with your arms extended, your hands beneath your shoulders, and your legs extended and your feet flexed. Keep your abs tight (A). Bend your left leg out to the side and bring your knee toward your left elbow (B). Pause, then return to the starting position. Switch sides. Do 20 reps, alternating sides.

Tone your upper chest to look great in sleeveless tops.

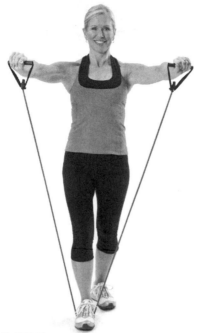

CRANK THE WHEEL

Stand with the band under one foot and hold an end in each hand. Extend your arms straight out in front of you at shoulder height. Don't lock your elbows. Rotate your hands in a circular motion, as if drawing circles with your fists. Do 10 reps in one direction. Repeat in the opposite direction.

I DID IT!

"My clothes look better and my body feels tighter."

—Kathy Melnychuk, 44; lost 3 pounds and 1¼ inches around her chest

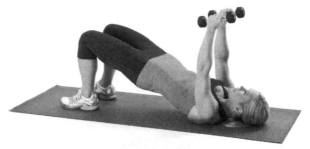

CHEST FLY WITH A BRIDGE

Hold dumbbells and lie faceup, with your knees bent, your feet flat, and your arms out to the sides (palms up, elbows slightly bent). Lift your hips so that your body forms a straight line from your knees to your shoulders. Squeeze your chest and raise your arms over your chest as though you're hugging a beach ball. Pause, and then slowly lower your arms. Keep your hips lifted throughout. Do 12 to 15 reps.

MELT SPILLOVER FAT

Our toning moves will firm up the muscles under those spillover spots. But to fully erase the bumps and bulges, you need to burn off excess fat as well, and that means cardio. Here's what we suggest to see the speediest results.

For under-arm flab and back fat, try:

• Cardio kickboxing: Tossing punches and jabs is a super trouble-spot firmer.
• Rowing machine: All those arm pulls are particularly good for shedding back fat.
• Swimming: Doing laps, especially the breaststroke, works the entire armpit area front and back.

For a muffin top, try:

• Zumba: This hot dance trend engages your abs while you shake your hips to shimmy off that unwanted belly roll.
• Water aerobics: Twisting and turning moves target and firm your waistline.
• Tennis: Every swing tones your abs and obliques.

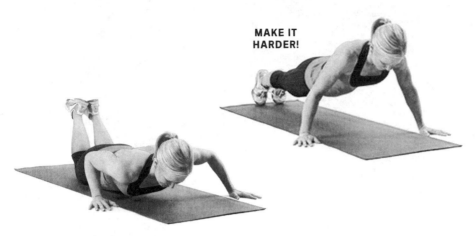

OFFSET PUSHUP

Begin on your hands (more than shoulder-width apart) and your knees so that your body forms a straight line from your head to your knees. Bend your elbows—the left one out to the side and the right one so it's close to your body—and lower your chest almost to the floor. Press back up and repeat on the other side, bending your right elbow out and keeping your left one in. Do 12 reps, alternating sides.

Make it harder: Extend your legs so that you're on your toes instead of your knees.

CHAPTER 16

The Belly Blaster

Get fit and firm faster—and lose up to two sizes—
with these miracle moves that triple results!

So you've lost some weight and toned some trouble spots. That's great! But maybe still your belly is poufier than you'd like. You've turned to the right page: You can blast belly fat faster than you ever believed possible with this turbo-charged plan that's guaranteed to melt fat and slash inches—in less than 30 minutes a day.

The secret: 3-in-1 toning moves that pair resistance bands with dumbbells. Research shows that this killer combo builds strength three times faster than standard-issue dumbbell exercises alone. But we didn't stop there. To speed your slim-down, we've added calorie-torching walking intervals and a waist-whittling eating plan (see page 218). A few times a week, you'll also do 20 to 30 minutes of whichever type of exercise you like best.

We know this approach works because we asked exercise scientists to test the program on 12 real women for 2 months. They got stronger and shapelier, and they lost up to 6 pounds in 3 weeks and up to 11 pounds by the end of the program.

THE PLAN AT A GLANCE

This plan combines Triple-Duty Toners (resistance band + dumbbell moves tighten three times faster) with Fat-Blast Intervals (quickie, high-intensity walking workouts burn through stubborn belly fat) plus Your-Choice Cardio (moderate-intensity exercise—the type you like best—fast-tracks weight loss) to melt away your middle.

YOUR BELLY BLAST-OFF PLAN

ACTIVITY	WEEK 1	WEEKS 2 AND 3	WEEKS 4 AND 5	WEEKS 6 AND 8
Triple-Duty Toners	1 set (bands only) 2 times per week	2 or 3 sets (bands only) 2 or 3 times per week	2 or 3 sets 2 or 3 times per week	2 or 3 sets 2 or 3 times per week
Fat-Blast Intervals	(None)	26 minutes 1 time per week	26 minutes 2 times per week	26 minutes 2 or 3 times per week
Your-Choice Cardio	20 minutes 2 or 3 times per week	30 minutes 2 times per week	30 minutes 1 time per week	30 minutes 1 time per week (optional)

Do 8 to 12 repetitions of each move to complete 1 set. (For the first 3 weeks, use bands only, then add dumbbells.) Once you get comfortable with the moves, work on increasing to 2 or 3 sets per workout, up to 3 times a week. For each exercise, the combined resistance of the dumbbell weight and the band strength should allow you to complete 8 reps to start. When you feel like you can keep going after 12 reps, increase the dumbbell weight, the resistance band strength, or both. If the band is too long, wrap it around your hand until it's the right length for you.

What you'll need: Light- to medium-weight dumbbells (3 to 8 pounds) and a flat 5- to 6-foot resistance band. Need bands? Find them at spri.com.

TRIPLE-DUTY CHEERLEADER PRESS
TARGETS SHOULDERS, BACKS OF ARMS

Stand with the band under your left foot, with the free end plus 1 dumbbell in your left hand. Bend your left elbow and raise your arm to chest level. This is the starting position (A). Press up (B). Bend your left elbow to lower your forearm behind you. Straighten, and then return to the starting position. That is 1 rep. Complete reps. Repeat on the opposite side for 1 set.

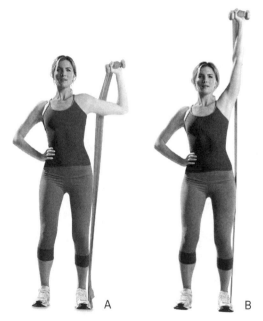

A   B

I DID IT!

"I've always hated shorts, but I just went out and bought two new pairs of Bermudas!"

—Lisa McCutcheon, 49; lost 6 pounds and gained 33 percent more leg strength in 8 weeks

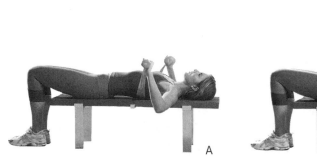 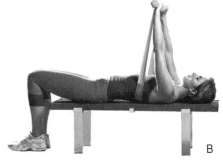

TRIPLE-DUTY CHEST PRESS
TARGETS CHEST, ARMS

Lie on a bench (a coffee table, a step bench, or the floor also works) faceup, with your knees bent and your feet flat on the floor, with the band under your back. Hold 1 end of the band plus 1 dumbbell in each hand, with your elbows bent and your hands near your chest (A). Press up until your arms are straight (B). Pause, then slowly return to the starting position.

TRIPLE-DUTY SQUAT AND CURL

Stand with your feet hip-width apart, with the middle of the band under both of your feet, 1 loose end plus 1 dumbbell in each hand, with your palms facing your sides. Bend your knees and lower as if you're sitting into a chair, keeping your knees behind your toes (A). Bend your elbows to curl your forearms upward, rotating your wrists so your palms face your chest, and pressing into your heels to stand (B). Slowly lower your arms back to the starting position.

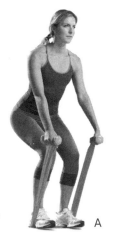 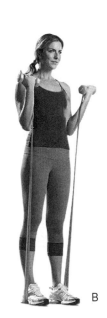

Get even more from your move! Balance on 1 leg as you squat, with the band under your standing foot. Switch the standing foot after each set.

TRIPLE-DUTY SKATER SIDE TWIST
TARGETS BUTT, HIPS, THIGHS, WAIST

Tie the band to the leg of a piece of heavy furniture. Stand with the anchored band to your left. Grasp the ends of the band and 1 dumbbell in both of your hands. Step diagonally back and to the left with your right foot, and bend both of your knees about 45 degrees as though you're going into a curtsy (A). Straighten your legs, bringing your right leg parallel to your left leg, and then rotate your torso to the right (B). Complete the reps. Repeat on the opposite side for 1 set.

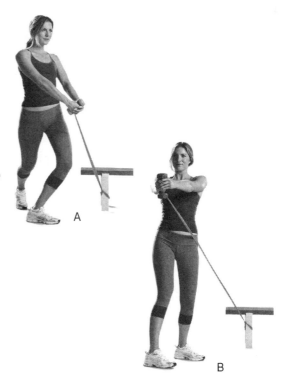

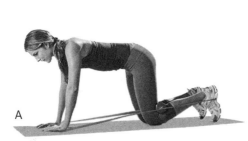

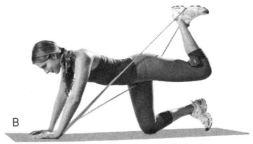

TRIPLE-DUTY BUTT KICKER
TARGETS BUTT, BACKS OF THIGHS, ABS

Get on your hands and knees, with your wrists below your shoulders and your knees below your hips. Wrap the band around your left heel and place a dumbbell in the crook of your left knee. Grasp 1 end of the band in each hand (A). Keeping your right foot flexed, press your left heel up and back (B). Lower to starting position. Complete reps. Repeat on the opposite side for 1 set.

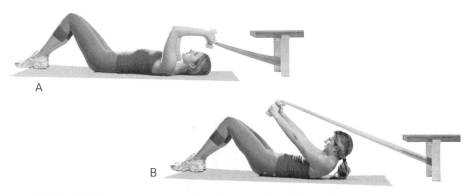

A

B

TRIPLE-DUTY PULLOVER AND CRUNCH
TARGETS ABS, BACKS OF ARMS

Tie the band to the leg of a piece of heavy furniture. Lie on your back with your head resting on the floor in front of the anchored band, with your knees bent. Bending your elbows, reach back to grasp 1 end of the band, along with 1 dumbbell, in each hand, with your arms bent about 90 degrees (A). Engage your abs to crunch upward. Staying lifted, press the weights forward, straightening your arms (B). Slowly lower your body, then your arms.

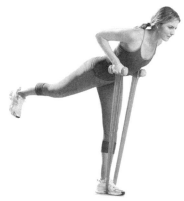

TRIPLE-DUTY BENT-OVER ROW
TARGETS BUTT, BACK, ARMS

Stand with your feet staggered, with your left foot in front. Place the middle of the band under your left foot and grasp 1 end of the band along with 1 dumbbell in each hand. Hinge forward and extend your right leg straight back until your torso and right leg are about parallel with the floor, with your arms hanging straight down. Bend your elbows to pull the band and dumbbells toward your underarms. Complete the reps, keeping your right leg lifted. Alternate the standing leg for each set.

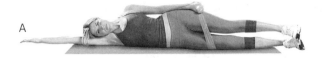

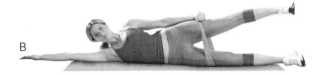

TRIPLE-DUTY SIDE LEG-LIFT CRUNCH
TARGETS BUTT, HIPS, WAIST

Wrap the band several times around the middle of 1 dumbbell, and then tie the remainder of the band around your thighs at arm's distance. Lie on your right side, with your legs stacked, your right arm extended, and your head resting on your arm. Rest the dumbbell on your left hip (A). Raise your left leg, crunching your torso a few inches off of the floor (B). Complete the reps. Repeat on your opposite side for 1 set.

 ——————————————————————————————

*"I was already a runner and biker,
but my legs have never looked this good!"*

—Merry Buckley, 39; lost 11 pounds and 6½ inches in 8 weeks

BUT WAIT, THERE'S MORE

This program was adapted from the book *Tone Every Inch* (Rodale, 2012), by Natalie Gingerich Mackenzie with the editors of *Prevention*. To pick up a copy of the full plan, go to toneeveryinch.com/pv.

YOUR FIRM-FASTER FOOD FORMULA!

Want to speed up your results? Design your own meals around these daily guidelines.

Breakfast: 300 calories with at least 8 grams of fiber and 20 grams of protein

Lunch: 300 calories with at least 8 grams of fiber and 20 grams of protein

Snack: 200 calories with at least 2 grams of fiber and 15 grams of protein

Dinner: 400 calories with at least 8 grams of fiber and 20 grams of protein

Snack: 200 calories with at least 2 grams of fiber and 15 grams of protein

Limit daily sodium intake to 2,300 milligrams. Look up the nutritional content of your favorite foods at nal.usda.gov/fnic/foodcomp/search.

FAT-BLAST INTERVALS

Want to shorten your workout time and get even better results? Alternate bursts of power walking with ones at a slowed-down pace. It increases the number of your mitochondria, the powerhouses in cells that convert fat to energy. The result: You burn more calories, even while you sleep. Here's your fat-blast interval workout. Gauge your effort level on a scale of 1 to 10: "1" is sitting on the couch; "10" is sprinting as hard as you can. For the intervals, alternate between 1 minute at an effort level of 7 to 8 followed by 1 minute at an effort level of 5 to 6. The total workout takes 26 minutes.

ACTIVITY	TIME	EFFORT LEVEL
Warmup	5 minutes	4 to 5
Intervals	19 minutes	Alternate
Cooldown	2 minutes	4 to 5

FIVE NEW WAYS TO BEAT BLOAT

Want to fit into your pants? Look at the carbs you're eating, says Jacqueline Wolf, MD, associate professor of medicine at Harvard Medical School and author of *A Woman's Guide to a Healthy Stomach*. Many are high in one of five hard-to-digest sugars: lactose, fructose, fructans, sugar alcohols, and galactans. To help relieve your symptoms, study your diet and follow these tips.

Stop milking it. If dairy makes you bloated, you might have developed lactose intolerance. Try lower-lactose foods (such as hard cheese or yogurt) or lactose-free dairy products, or take a lactase enzyme.

Pick fruit carefully. Berries, grapes, and citrus contain a near-equal ratio of the sugars fructose and glucose, making them easier to digest than fruits with more fructose, such as honeydew, apples, and pears.

Switch your starch. If fructan-rich wheat, rye, or barley is behind your bloat, choose stomach-friendly rice, corn, oats, or potatoes.

Skip (some) fake sugars. Is your gum blowing you up? Sorbitol, xylitol, and mannitol are sugar alcohols found in diet sodas and sugar-free gum. Avoid these if they bother you, or opt for products made with stevia or aspartame instead.

Be smart about beans. Limit galactan-rich legumes (soy nuts, chickpeas, lentils, and all beans), cabbage, and Brussels sprouts if they're causing you trouble. Soaking dried beans overnight or taking the over-the-counter enzyme Beano might help.

Part 4

NUTRITION
NEWS

CHAPTER 17

A Good Egg

What really matters—and doesn't—when it comes to buying eggs? To find out, we visited working farms. What we learned may scramble everything you thought you knew about the Incredible, Edible Egg.

Glance down at that fresh egg in the carton, and what do you see? A versatile food and a near-perfect capsule of energy and protein? Or a stealthy delivery system for Salmonella bacteria?

If you chose the latter, it's probably because you remember the August 2010 *Salmonella Enteritidis* outbreak, which prompted the recall of more than 500 million eggs after nearly 2,000 people became sick with fever, abdominal cramps, and diarrhea.

In the aftermath of the outbreak, disturbing reports emerged about the two Iowa companies that produced the tainted eggs—Wright County Egg and Hillandale Farms, both of which were shut down by the FDA until they could remedy the problems. The government pinned the blame on Salmonella contamination throughout the henhouses, in both the chicken feed and droppings. But FDA inspectors also found mice, flies, and wild birds indoors, and hens that had escaped from their cages and were wandering through immense piles of manure. None of this did anything to improve the image of big commercial egg farms, which had already been criticized for squeezing hens into tiny, restrictive cages.

In the months after the Great Egg Scare, producers of organic, cage-free, and free-range eggs struggled to keep up with a sudden surge in consumer demand. But while there is much to recommend those eggs—including a ban on toxic pesticides and genetically modified organisms (GMOs) in the hens' feed—an ironclad guarantee that they are Salmonella free is not one of the advantages. According to public health officials, the main thing that keeps eggs germ free is how an individual farmer—whether conventional or organic—manages a hen's eggs at every stage of the process, from laying to washing, packing, and transporting.

Prevention visited three farms—one conventional, one large-scale organic, and one small, local organic—for a firsthand glimpse of the journey of an egg from the hen to your plate.

Prepare to be surprised.

THE CONVENTIONAL FARM

The 100-acre conventional farm owned by Elmer Martin lies in the lush, rolling Pennsylvania Dutch countryside of Lancaster County. Before mounting the stairs to the henhouse door, visitors must don disposable coveralls—zipped-up, full-body protective suits of a thin polyester, finished with plastic booties—which makes this tour feel a little like an adventure into a Hot Zone virus lab. The protection is not for the visitors, though; it's for the birds. Outsiders could easily introduce dangerous foreign bacteria and contaminants on their clothes and shoes.

Martin's henhouse is a long, narrow, windowless, industrial-looking building set off on a patch of bright green grass. We walk through the door and into a large, open, dim space that stretches 450 feet (the length of 1½ football fields) and houses 87,000 birds—a little less than a typical henhouse on a factory farm. Wooden walkways stretch into the dusty distance between rows of cages, which are stacked four high. Hens are housed, in groups of seven, in cages that measure 20 by 24 inches—yielding each bird a space smaller than the size of an 8½- by 11-inch piece of paper. The air is acrid and filled with the cluckings and shufflings of thousands of birds. They screech when we approach, but there's not enough room for them even to flap their wings.

WHAT'S IN A CLAIM?

Any carton of eggs you buy is likely to be plastered with descriptive terms. Some are meaningful, but others are misleading.

CERTIFIED HUMANE-RAISED AND HANDLED: Meets the standards of the Humane Farm Animal Care program, which is an independent nonprofit. The standards include being cage free and having sufficient space to engage in natural behaviors such as dust bathing and perching.

UNITED EGG PRODUCERS CERTIFIED: The eggs were produced in compliance with industry-codified standard practices. (More than 80 percent of commercial eggs carry this seal.)

ALL-NATURAL: The hens eat vegetarian feed, with no animal slaughterhouse by-products.

CAGE FREE: Hens must live in an open space, not a cage or a coop, but the "open space" can be inside a crowded henhouse. Both organic and conventional hens can be cage free.

FREE-RANGE: Similar to cage free, except that birds have some degree of outdoor access—though the amount, duration, or quality of that outdoor time is not specified.

PASTURE-RAISED: Hens are allowed to range on fresh pasture. Often they are housed in trailers that can be towed to different fields.

ORGANIC: Hens must be given organic feed, which contains no toxic pesticides, herbicides, or fungicides and no GMOs or slaughterhouse by-products. They must never be caged, and they must have outdoor access. The USDA certifies this designation.

The hens spend their productive years in these cages, pecking at the feed that shuttles past in an automatic trough and laying their eggs—about five per week—which roll down the sloped floor of the cage to another trough that carries them into the next room for cooling and storing. Most of the hens never even get to ogle a rooster, because they lay eggs whether or not a male is in the vicinity. When they are too old to produce "good" eggs, at around 24 months of age, they're shipped out to be slaughtered for various cooked-chicken products such as canned chicken meat.

As unsettling as the scene may be to a newcomer, Martin's farm is at the forefront of egg safety because it participates in the Pennsylvania Egg Quality Assurance Program (PEQAP), which has made strides against Salmonella by controlling risk factors, according to Paul H. Patterson, PhD, professor of poultry science at Pennsylvania State University in University Park, one of PEQAP's founders. The Pennsylvania program has been so effective that its methods served as the basis of a mandatory new set of FDA guidelines, called the Egg Safety Rule, which began being phased in across the country in 2010—though not in time to prevent the Iowa outbreaks.

As part of PEQAP, Martin buys only chicks that have been certified Salmonella free, and he tests them again before bringing them into the henhouse. For added assurance, he regularly monitors the barn for any trace of the bacteria by dragging swabs through manure pits under the cages and then sending samples to state labs to test for any trace of the germs. And he cleans out the manure at least once a month—versus as seldom as once every 2 years at some conventional facilities. Equally important, Martin takes multiple measures to keep out rats, mice, flies, and wild birds, which can spread Salmonella bacteria around the henhouse.

The Pennsylvania system has proven that eggs from conventional caged hens can be made very low risk. In 1992, when the program began, 26 percent of the manure samples that inspectors took from participating Pennsylvania henhouses tested positive for Salmonella. Now it's down to 1 percent.

"We believe the Egg Safety Rule, once fully implemented nationally in 5 to 10 years, can help prevent roughly 79,000 illnesses annually," says Don Kraemer, acting deputy director for operations at the FDA's Center for Food Safety and Applied Nutrition. That would represent a reduction of more than 50 percent from the current FDA estimate of 142,000 egg-borne Salmonella cases a year.

THE ORGANIC FARM

Just down the road from Elmer Martin is Robert Keller's farm. It has all the advantages of a PEQAP farm but, in addition, it's organic. Organic operations have a much higher level of oversight than conventional farms do. To maintain their certification and use the organic seal on their product, farms have to be inspected annually, at a minimum, by a third-party certifier with USDA accreditation. Compare that with the sporadic oversight of conventional facilities by the FDA, which has been chronically strapped for resources.

"The FDA had never conducted a routine inspection of one of the farms involved in last year's big recall," says Patty Lovera, assistant director of Food & Water Watch, a nonprofit in Washington, DC, dedicated to safe and sustainable food practices.

That doesn't mean that organic operations necessarily conform to the bucolic images that most people have in mind. In fact, most supermarket "organic" eggs are produced in factory-size facilities. The producers follow the letter of the National Organic Program, which requires that the poultry receive organic feed, are cage free, and have "outdoor access." There isn't, however, any mandate about how much time the chickens need to spend in the great outdoors.

Keller's 23,800 birds live in a 450-foot-long henhouse with three tiers of perches; they're indoors in inclement weather but otherwise often outdoors by day, exiting by portals. They have more than three times more space per bird than Martin's hens, but the barn is still crowded. Most of the birds mill about on the floor, with some of them—those higher up in the pecking order—perching on the less-crowded upper levels. Most of the hens lay their eggs in the darkened nesting boxes.

Over the past 5 years, multiple studies, including one massive survey of 23 European countries, have shown lower rates of Salmonella in cage-free hens (both organic and conventional). Experts believe that's largely a function of smaller flocks, making sanitary conditions easier to maintain.

"Organic farmers aren't allowed to use antibiotics or most other drugs to treat their flocks," says Mark Kastel, cofounder of the Cornucopia Institute in Cornucopia, Wisconsin, a pro-organic group. "It's incumbent on them to create a healthier environment."

Organic feed is also less vulnerable to contamination. Conventional "chicken mash" is based on corn and soy, but it can also include slaughterhouse waste, which may be tainted with any of the germs that infected the animals themselves, says Michael Greger, MD, director of public health and animal agriculture at the Humane Society of the United States in Washington, DC. By contrast, organic feed cannot contain by-products from mammals or poultry.

"And safety isn't only about pathogens that can land you in the hospital," says Kastel. "Organic feed is also free of toxic pesticides, herbicides, and fungicides and contains no genetically modified organisms."

HANDLED WITH CARE

Prevention has a 60-year interest in healthy and safe farming techniques. The magazine's owners and founders, the Rodale family, have been committed to studying and promoting the links between organic farming and healthy soil, healthy food, and healthy people since the 1940s through the Rodale Institute in Kutztown, Pennsylvania.

In addition, the family's own farm in Allentown, Pennsylvania, includes 90-some laying chickens, which are "allowed to be chickens," says Maya Rodale, great-granddaughter of company founder J.I. Rodale. The Rodale hens have daily access to fresh pasture outside the stone building that houses them, eat organic feed, and wander back to the laying boxes when they're ready to produce an egg. At night, they roost on 2-foot-tall perches in the middle of the house, where they naturally flock for safety. The eggs they produce feed the Rodale family and are also used at the Rodale cafeterias. Any surplus is given to Second Harvest, a local food pantry.

THE SMALL, LOCAL ORGANIC FARM

To many proponents of sustainable food, however, the most desirable eggs come from smaller, local organic farms. These are much closer to what a conscientious shopper probably envisions when she picks up a dozen "cage-free" eggs at the market. And it's the life that the 150 chickens at the 20-acre Neversink Farm in the foothills of New York's Catskill Mountains enjoy, nestled amid wooded hills, fields of flowers, and a pond full of trout. At this small organic farm—established by Conor and Katie Crickmore 1 ½ years ago—the birds have a small, rounded coop that they can leave and return to at will, restrained only by a movable electric fence that keeps them in—and predators out.

The birds at Neversink Farm are "pasture-raised"—meaning the hens are moved to a different patch of land every day when the fence posts are shifted, allowing the chickens to hunt and peck for a new crop of grass and insects in addition to their certified organic feed, which the Crickmores grind themselves, so it is always fresh.

On our arrival, instead of screeching and cowering like caged birds, the hens cluck and circle our feet in curiosity. When one strays too far, Conor picks it up and cradles it. He describes the different chicken sounds a farmer learns to recognize. There's a squawking "complaining sound" that often means "I want corn," as opposed to the singsongy sound the hens make when they're foraging. Both are different from the "egg-laying" sound, which is a loud caw. And the birds coo themselves to sleep.

Because the flock is so small, Neversink Farm is not required to follow the FDA's Egg Safety Rule, which exempts producers with fewer than 3,000 birds. (As a certified organic farm, it is bound by the National Organic Program.) But the Crickmores are so confident of the safety of their product that they consume their own eggs raw in homemade mayonnaise. With a small flock and ample space, manure management is not a major problem. Conor and Katie scatter a new layer of straw on the floor of the coop every day, protecting the birds from their excrement and allowing the manure to dry for composting later. In spring and summer, it will be used to fertilize their vegetable fields.

Being out in the fields and not crowded into tight quarters, the hens don't spread infections as quickly as caged hens do, and farmers say they develop healthier immune systems this way. The birds can also engage in their natural behaviors, including "dust bathing," which cleans their feathers, says Honor Schauland, campaign assistant for the Organic Consumers Association, who raises chickens for eggs on her farm in northeastern Minnesota.

Research suggests that pasture-raised eggs may even have superior nutritional content. Scientists at Pennsylvania State University found 2½ times more omega-3s and twice the vitamin E in the eggs of pasture-raised hens (which were given feed as a supplement to their forage) than those of caged hens that were fed only standard commercial mash.

"Leafy plants like grasses, white clover, red clover, alfalfa, and legumes contain more vitamins and unsaturated fatty acids than standard mash does," says Heather Karsten, PhD, associate professor of crop and soil sciences at Penn State, who conducted the study. (Some producers of both organic and conventional eggs enrich their hens' feed to boost omega-3s or other nutrients.)

So, which eggs are safest? The issue is highly contentious among poultry experts. Claims and counterclaims ping-pong back and forth between the opposing camps. Some commercial producers contend that cleanliness can be a greater challenge in cage-free facilities, because the birds mill around at the bottom of the henhouse, stepping in each other's excrement. And birds that range outside, they say, can pick up PCBs or other contaminants from the soil.

Organic producers counter with research showing that the fewer birds per henhouse, the lower the risks.

"Cage-free and organic flocks are, by definition, smaller because you can't fit as many into the henhouse," says Dr. Greger at the Humane Society.

Does this mean that organic eggs are 100 percent safe? No. Vigilance and enforcement are still farm-by-farm initiatives. If any egg producers fail to keep rats and mice out of their farms—or if they buy infected flocks to begin with—those eggs might be tainted.

In general, though, the risks of infection in both organic and conventional eggs remain low. The CDC and food scientists estimate that, nationally, only 1 in 20,000 eggs is contaminated.

"You could literally eat raw eggs for 60 years and never encounter one that is positive for Salmonella," says Kevin M. Keener, PhD, professor of food science and food process engineer at Purdue University in West Lafayette, Indiana. But if you should be one of the unlucky ones to ingest a Salmonella-tainted egg, the consequences could be fever and upset stomach—or hospitalization and even death, particularly among the very young or very old.

That's why we all have a stake in industry practices that will give us a good egg.

CHAPTER 18

A Better Burger

Break away from ground beef with mouthwatering makeovers of everyone's favorite. Try our flavorful toppings and sauces to give these healthy burgers a boost.

Burgers might be basic, but they don't have to be boring. The following delicious, nutritious recipes replace ground beef with other healthful, unusual ingredients, such as mushrooms, crab, bison, chicken, and salmon. The nutrition information that you'll find here is for the recipes as written, but you should feel free to mix and match and be inspired. For example, you could try the crab cakes on the pita or the chicken sliders on mini buns.

For the best burgers, don't flip your burger before its time. If it's sticking to the grill or pan, it hasn't browned enough to seal in the juices, so it's not ready to turn. And avoid the temptation to press down on the patties with your spatula. All this does is dries them out.

WILD MUSHROOM-LENTIL BURGERS

Makes 4 servings

6 ounces shiitake mushrooms

1 can (15½ ounces) lentils, rinsed and drained

¾ cup fresh whole wheat bread crumbs (from 1 slice)

1 large egg

¼ cup chopped celery

1½ tablespoons fresh thyme

2 teaspoons Dijon mustard

1 cup chopped onion, divided

4 ounces mild goat cheese, divided

6 tablespoons fine yellow cornmeal

3 teaspoons olive oil, divided

4 whole wheat buns, toasted

¼ cup chopped roasted red bell peppers

¼ cup watercress

Heat the oven to 400°F.

Remove the stems from the mushrooms and discard. Coarsely chop three-quarters of the mushroom caps and put in a food processor. Quarter the remaining mushroom caps and set aside.

Add the lentils, bread crumbs, egg, celery, thyme, mustard, ½ cup of the onion, and 2 ounces of the cheese to the food processor. Pulse until coarsely chopped. Form into 4 patties (3" diameter). Put the cornmeal on a plate and gently coat the patties on all sides (patties will be very delicate).

Heat 1 teaspoon of the oil in a large nonstick skillet over medium heat. Add the reserved mushrooms and the remaining ½ cup onion and cook until the onion is golden, 5 to 6 minutes. Remove from the pan and set aside.

Add the remaining 2 teaspoons oil to the pan and cook the patties, turning once, until golden brown, about 6 minutes. Transfer to a baking sheet, top with the remaining 2 ounces cheese, and bake until heated through, about 4 minutes.

Serve the burgers on the buns and top with the reserved mushroom mixture, peppers, and watercress.

PER SERVING: 386 calories, 19 g protein, 51 g carbohydrates, 13 g total fat, 6 g saturated fat, 12 g fiber, 597 mg sodium

Note: Lentils are rich in fiber and folate and make this meatless meal especially heart-smart.

CRAB CAKE BURGERS
WITH REMOULADE SAUCE

Makes 4 servings

½ pound lump crabmeat

1 large egg white

⅜ teaspoon ground black pepper, divided

1½ cups panko bread crumbs, divided

½ cup reduced-fat mayonnaise, divided

2 shallots, finely chopped and divided

2 tablespoons fresh lemon juice, divided

2 tablespoons chopped fresh tarragon, divided

2 tablespoons chopped fresh chives, divided

4 multigrain buns, toasted

¼ cup radish sprouts

Heat the oven to 400°F.

Combine the crabmeat, egg white, ¼ teaspoon of the pepper, ½ cup of the panko, ¼ cup of the mayonnaise, half of the shallots, and 1 tablespoon each of the lemon juice, tarragon, and chives. Form into 4 patties and coat in remaining 1 cup panko.

Mix remaining ⅛ teaspoon pepper and remaining ¼ cup mayonnaise, shallots, and 1 tablespoon each lemon juice, tarragon, and chives in a small bowl for sauce.

Brown the patties in a nonstick pan coated with cooking spray over medium heat, 2 minutes per side. Put on a baking sheet. Bake until heated through, about 4 minutes.

Serve on the buns and top with the sauce and sprouts.

PER SERVING: 348 calories, 20 g protein, 36 g carbohydrates, 14 g total fat, 3 g saturated fat, 2 g fiber, 683 mg sodium

Note: Using reduced-fat mayonnaise cuts 100 calories from each burger.

BBQ CHICKEN SLIDERS

Makes 6 servings

1 small red onion

1 pound ground chicken

$\frac{1}{2}$ cup chopped cilantro + 6 sprigs

$\frac{3}{4}$ teaspoon cumin

6 tablespoons barbecue sauce, divided

2 whole wheat pitas

6 thin slices smoked Gouda ($\frac{3}{4}$ ounce total)

Chop half of the onion to measure $\frac{1}{4}$ cup and slice the remaining half.

Combine the chopped onion, chicken, chopped cilantro, cumin, and 4 tablespoons of the barbecue sauce. Form into 6 equal (3" diameter) patties (mixture will be very wet).

Separate pitas and cut each half with a 3" round cookie cutter to make 12 circles.

Heat a lightly oiled grill to medium heat. Grill the burgers for 4 minutes, turn, and top with the cheese. Grill until cooked through, about 5 minutes longer.

Serve each burger between pita rounds with sliced onion, cilantro sprigs, and 1 teaspoon of the remaining barbecue sauce.

PER SERVING: 210 calories, 16 g protein, 20 g carbohydrates, 8 g total fat, 3 g saturated fat, 2 g fiber, 386 mg sodium

Note: Smoked Gouda is extra flavorful so you can use less.

TASTY TOPPERS

Design your own burger with these out-of-the-ordinary flavor enhancers. They're all easy to find in your supermarket's ethnic foods section, olive bar, condiment aisle, and produce and prepared foods departments.

GRILLED OR ROASTED VEGGIES: tomatoes, onions, zucchini, radicchio, or peppers

CHUTNEYS: tomato, mango, or cranberry

PESTOS: cilantro, basil, or arugula

DIPS: guacamole, salsa, or hummus

PICKLED VEGGIES: onions, okra, jalapeños, carrots, pepperoncini, or kimchi

HOT SAUCES: harissa, chipotle chiles in adobo sauce, sambal oelek, or Sriracha

SLAWS: broccoli, carrot, or cabbage

BISON BURGERS

Makes 4 servings

1 pound ground bison or buffalo, preferably grass fed

2 teaspoons Worcestershire sauce

6 tablespoons hot-pepper jelly, divided

4 thin slices 2% milk Cheddar cheese (1 ounce total)

3 tomatoes, sliced

Combine the bison or buffalo, Worcestershire, and 2 tablespoons of the jelly. Form into 4 equal (3½" diameter) patties.

Heat a lightly oiled grill to medium heat. Grill the burgers for 4 minutes, turn, and top with the cheese. Grill 3 to 4 minutes longer for medium-rare. Let the burgers stand for 5 minutes.

Serve the burgers with the tomatoes and the remaining 4 tablespoons jelly.

PER SERVING: 254 calories, 25 g protein, 18 g carbohydrates, 10 g total fat, 4 g saturated fat, 1 g fiber, 217 mg sodium

Note: Grass-fed ground bison is pricier than the grain-fed kind but worth it—it's lower in calories and fat. Serve this bunless burger with tomato slices.

ASIAN SALMON BURGERS

Makes 4 servings

1 pound skinless salmon fillet, cut into chunks

¼ cup fresh whole wheat bread crumbs

1 large egg white

2 large cloves garlic, chopped

2 teaspoons reduced-sodium soy sauce

½ teaspoon dark sesame oil

2 scallions, chopped

4 tablespoons pickled ginger, divided

2 tablespoons toasted sesame seeds

4 whole wheat buns, toasted

¼ cup baby spinach

Put the salmon, bread crumbs, egg white, garlic, soy sauce, oil, scallions, and 2 tablespoons of the ginger in a food processor. Pulse until coarsely chopped. Form into 4 equal (3" diameter) patties. Sprinkle the tops with the sesame seeds.

Heat a large nonstick skillet coated with cooking spray over medium heat. Put the patties sesame-seed-side down in the pan. Cook for 5 minutes. Turn and cook until done, 5 minutes longer.

Serve the burgers on the buns and top with the spinach and the remaining 2 tablespoons pickled ginger.

PER SERVING: 426 calories, 30 g protein, 29 g carbohydrates, 21 g total fat, 4 g saturated fat, 5 g fiber, 501 mg sodium

Note: Pickled ginger adds taste and visual appeal for only 5 calories per tablespoon.

CHAPTER 19

The New Vegetarian

These four women walked away from meat for different reasons—and say doing so changed their lives for the better. Could it change yours?

Shortly after giving up meat in 1995, Jessica Lindsey took a cross-country trip that gave her a taste of what eating out was going to be like.

"Vegetarianism was still so fringe then that hardly anyone outside of California knew what it meant," she says. "At one restaurant, the waitress told me that the soups were vegetarian. She said that the broth was from beef, and it contained chicken pieces, but no meat!"

Today, Lindsey rarely has such strange encounters. Vegetarianism is steadily becoming mainstream. Roughly 6 to 8 million Americans are vegetarians, according to the Vegetarian Resource Group—up from a half million to 2 million in 1994. And they've gotten smarter about their dining choices. A generation ago, vegetarian meals were often built around leaden nut loaves or uninspired brown-rice casseroles. Today, many vegetarians consider themselves

THE MEATLESS MONDAY MOVEMENT

If you don't think you can commit to going totally meatless, try 1 day a week. The Meatless Monday campaign has taken off recently, with high-profile chefs such as Mario Batali and John Fraser adding meatless specials to their popular restaurants' Monday night menus. "Mondays used to be slow nights for us," says Fraser, who owns the three-star Dovetail in New York City. "Now we're booked solid."

Find four new veggie recipes every week at meatlessmonday.com.

foodies and relish the challenge of finding recipes that showcase fresh vegetables as a delicious main course, flavored with herbs and spices.

"Vegetables are becoming culinary rock stars," says Amanda Cohen, owner of the vegetarian restaurant Dirt Candy in New York City.

As these four women show, there are many potential benefits to eating vegetarian. Read on . . .

THE ORGANIC GARDENER

Susan Kayne, 44, of Hudson, New York, is a horse breeder who's married with a grown daughter. Susan has been a vegetarian for 10 years and a vegan for 6 months. Here's her story.

"At this time of year, all the vegetables I eat I grow myself in my large organic garden—heirloom tomatoes, zucchini, patty pan squash, carrots, basil, parsley, dill. Sure, it's cheaper and more delicious than store-bought veggies, but that only partially explains why I'm out there watering at 7:00 a.m. Growing your own food is so much better for your health and for the environment too.

"It's been a gradual process for me. I gave up meat 10 years ago strictly for health reasons. I was concerned about the hormones used in beef. Then 3 or 4 years ago, my daughter, Rachel, now 21, began giving me books on the environment. A couple of points really made an impact on me—like the fact that producing meat requires up to 50 times more fossil fuels than growing veggies, or that it takes four times more farmland to feed a meat eater for a year. Thanks to those books, I eliminated eggs and milk from my diet too.

"Now I'm purely vegan, and I eat more produce than I ever imagined possible. I'll sauté a big batch of veggies for the week. I freeze vegetables straight from my garden and can them, and I make my own salsa. Last year, I even treated myself to a spiral slicer that helps me make noodle-like strands from summer squash. When mixed with tomatoes, garlic, olive oil, and a little nutritional yeast, it's like heaven on a plate."

The Payoff

"Before I started packing my diet with fruits and vegetables, I used to gain weight easily. Now my scale steadily reads 135 (I'm 5-foot-9), and, much to my surprise, my body shape has changed. I don't have belly fat, and my hips and legs seem slimmer.

"But I'm most thrilled with my improved energy level. In the past, when I ate a lot of meat, I used to feel like going to sleep right after a meal, or else I'd get a burst of energy but crash an hour later. Now my energy level is steady. I never feel depleted, even after running a couple of miles around the neighborhood."

RAW OR COOKED?

You want to make the most of every delicious vegetarian bite. Although raw produce is often assumed to be more nutritious than cooked, a mix of both kinds gives you more healthy options.

TOMATOES: Cooked, these have a higher dose of cancer-fighting lycopene.

ZUCCHINI: Squash delivers more beta-carotene (a building block for vitamin A) when cooked.

SPINACH: Raw spinach has more vitamin C and folate. Cooked, it's richer in calcium and zinc.

GREEN BELL PEPPERS: You'll keep more B vitamins if you eat these raw.

GARLIC: Garlic's health-protecting antimicrobial power is dimmed by cooking.

THE HEART HEALER

Jessica Lindsey, 45, of San Francisco, is a collectibles dealer who's married with one child. She's been a vegetarian for 16 years. In her own words:

"My father rarely ate a healthy meal. He always had a big burger or a stack of saucy chicken wings. Still, when I got the call that he had passed away suddenly of a heart attack at age 54 (I was 24), I couldn't believe it. I knew that eating a lot of saturated fat caused heart trouble, but it never hit home before, even though both of my grandfathers had also died of heart attacks.

"In the weeks after Dad's funeral, I began to think about my own diet. The meats I loved—hot dogs, salami, bacon—were among the unhealthiest ones you could buy. I'd eat them with a side of starch—not whole grains, either—and I picked around any vegetables. Seriously, I ate like a 3-year-old. I figured I was doomed unless I did something drastic.

"That's when I decided to give up beef and pork. At first, I did it all wrong, replacing my hot dogs with pasta, my bacon with muffins, and my salami with more pasta. Friends would joke that I was a 'starchatarian.' But after my daughter, Sasha, was born in 2003, I vowed to learn to like veggies along with her. Mushrooms became a surprise favorite. At first, I'd just eat them on pizza, but then I began eating portobellos. Mmmm. I've also discovered that stir-frying

THE VEGETARIAN VARIETIES

The lingo can get complicated. A strict vegetarian doesn't eat any meat or animal-derived products, though some make exceptions for fish, dairy, or eggs. Here's a guide.

PESCATARIANS: eat fish

OVO-VEGETARIANS: eat eggs

LACTO-VEGETARIANS: eat dairy products

LACTO-PESCO-OVO VEGETARIANS: eat all three

VEGANS: eat no animals or animal products, including milk and honey

DON'T BE A "STARCHATARIAN"

When you go vegetarian, it's a common misstep to replace meat with starch. However, such a diet is no healthier than a meat-based diet and might even be less so. Instead, fill the empty spaces on your plate with plant-based protein—nuts, seeds, soy, and legumes contain plenty. In addition, aim to get enough of the following nutrients, which can fall short.

IRON: For nonmeat sources, turn to egg yolks, beans, and cooked spinach.

CALCIUM: Nondairy eaters should opt for leafy greens such as kale.

OMEGA-3S: If fish isn't on your menu, be sure to consume walnuts and flax-seed, and consider a supplement.

VITAMIN B_{12}: This nutrient occurs naturally only in animal products, so you must either supplement or eat fortified foods, such as cereals or soy milk.

cauliflower and bell peppers in olive oil and garlic does wonders for their flavor. It makes me feel good now when Sasha asks, 'Can I have more carrots, Mom?'"

The Payoff

"Though my cholesterol isn't as low as I'd like it to be (darn genes!), my doctor swears that if I'd kept my diet as it was, I'd be on medicine by now and a prime candidate for an early heart attack. Being vegetarian also helps me keep my weight steady. I'm 5-foot-6 and 132—about the same as 20 years ago."

THE ANIMAL ACTIVIST

Marsha Godzinski Hargreaves, 57, of Savannah, Georgia, is a registered nurse who's married with no children. She's been a vegan for 1 year. Here's her story, in her own words.

"Ever since childhood, I've been an animal lover. But it was only 4 years ago that I finally made the connection between what was in my heart and what was going into my mouth. There was no specific event that led to it. It just dawned on me that if I cared for animals as much as I said, I should boot beef, pork, and poultry from my diet.

"Then in January 2010, I became involved in the animal-rights movement. I participated in a protest outside a circus, and I saw a video of a baby elephant being taken from her mother by a trainer and tied to the ground. She was trembling. It upset me so much that I went home that night and threw out all the dairy, fish, and eggs in the fridge. I had no idea what to eat. I lived on vegan frozen dinners and protein bars for 3 months.

"My husband, Jim, supported my decision, but he didn't want any part of my new eating habits himself at first. He cooked his own food. We had separate cutting boards, utensils, and dishes. Then, as I learned more about vegan diets through cookbooks and blogs, I stopped buying processed products and started playing around in the kitchen again. One of the first vegan recipes I tried was lentil barley soup. Jim, who has always loved lentils, finished the leftovers before I could get to them. We have both enjoyed my homemade hummus and a whole wheat pasta dish with cabbage, peas, and beans. Interestingly, as I've backed off trying to get him to follow my diet, he's shown more interest. The other day, my bacon-and-eggs husband asked me to make him a veggie smoothie for breakfast!"

The Payoff

"Within 3 months of adopting a vegan diet, my total cholesterol plummeted 100 points. My doctor took me off my blood pressure medication about 6 months ago because she didn't think I would need it anymore. Every time I have my blood pressure checked, it's well within the normal range."

THE WEIGHT-LOSS WINNER

Laura Wooster Baldwin, 35, of Arlington, Virginia, is a marketing consultant who's married with no children. She's been a vegan for 2 ½ years. In her own words:

"The year after I got married, my weight jumped from 120 to 135, and those 15 pounds made a big difference on my 5-foot-3 frame. Although I wasn't pigging out on junk food, I didn't exactly have the healthiest diet. I rarely, if ever, ate vegetables. So I made a 2009 New Year's resolution: I'd try the popular Blue Print Cleanse for 4 days (drinking only fruit and vegetable juices), then cut all animal products out of my diet for the next 3 months.

"My British husband was not about to give up meat, but he was very supportive of my decision—so I cooked, and he ate. I made stews stuffed with chickpeas, tomatoes, and seitan (wheat gluten). I roasted onions, garlic, broccoli, peppers, and other veggies to bring out their sweetness. I found delicious soy-free vegan sausages, which I made with kale and polenta. I was loving the food—and the results. Three months passed, and I never looked back."

The Payoff

"I was back at my old weight of 120 pounds before my 3-month vegan trial ended, and I've held steady at 115 pounds for 2 ½ years. Before, I was a horrendous cook, but vegetables are a lot more forgiving than meats, so now I'm more confident in the kitchen. The best part is how I feel: Now that my meals consist of nutritious foods, I feel and look healthier all around."

BUT WAIT, THERE'S MORE

If you'd like to try these women's favorite vegetarian recipes, visit prevention.com/veggie-recipes.

CHAPTER 20

Mothers against Junk Dining

Out with processed chicken nuggets and in with whole-food feasts. A new generation of young families is rising up to the challenge!

"Eat your vegetables" is a joyless edict that's been uttered over sodden plates of greens for generations. But you won't hear that mantra around Christine di Palma's table. Her 5-year-old daughter, Marlie, clamors for vegetables, and she can also rattle off their nutritional highlights. Why? Di Palma has always made veggie-heavy dishes based on unprocessed ingredients the only option at her house.

Di Palma, 37, is hardly alone at the organic market. Best-selling books including Michael Pollan's *The Omnivore's Dilemma* and TV series such as *Jamie Oliver's Food Revolution* have changed the way many families think about food. A generation ago, packaged and frozen meals were celebrated as an escape from the drudgery of the kitchen. But now more moms have become educated and outspoken about using less-processed foods that are free of pesticides, food dyes, hormones, and antibiotics.

The challenge is balancing a desire to feed a family this way with the usual time demands and budget constraints. But the following moms have shown that it is possible. While they are the first to acknowledge that they're not perfect (Twinkies happen), their kids are growing up with a healthy suspicion of chicken nuggets and a serious vegetable tooth.

THE COST-CONSCIOUS COOK

Lisa Leake, 34, is a blogger in Charlotte, North Carolina.

Not long ago, Leake didn't stress about what her kids ate. She planned meals around coupons and sales. As for the cupboard filled with chips, cookies, and candies, well, those were just normal all-American snacks. It was only after she saw a TV interview in which food activist and author Michael Pollan discussed the pitfalls of the modern industrial diet that she took a hard look at what her family was eating.

Leake grew up on convenience foods, though her husband was "raised by organic hippies in Oregon." He might have fed the family differently, she says, but cooking was her job. When she changed her family's diet a year ago, she dragged him in and out of stores, mining his knowledge of the foods he ate as a kid.

In the process, Leake became a food expert herself. She now writes a blog, 100DaysofRealFood.com, to help others who want to rehab their own family diets.

The hardest part of the process for Leake was the resistance she faced from a 3-year-old and a 5-year-old who were too young to understand why Froot Loops were suddenly forbidden: "For a couple of weeks, they cried for Oreos." But Leake

ON THE MENU

Here's a sample menu at the Leake home.

BREAKFAST: Oatmeal with honey, cinnamon, and raisins

LUNCH: Egg salad on whole wheat with apples and grapes

DINNER: Quesadillas with chopped vegetables, cheese, and cilantro

never gave in. To pull off a transition like this, she says, parents must be role models. "You won't get away with hiding cookies on the top shelf," she says.

Leake eased the pain by providing organic versions of the things the kids loved, like a homemade pizza Lunchable. But now nuts, not Oreos, are a typical snack.

"Within a few weeks, there was a new normal," she says.

Blog readers complained that anyone could eat organic, given the unlimited food budget Leake seemed to have. So she pledged to limit spending to $125 a week to feed the family of four for 100 days.

Leake discovered she and her family can eat an organic diet without breaking the bank. After completing the challenge, she has settled on a budget of $150 per week, which is well within the typical household's reach. The USDA tracks food costs and reported that in April 2011, the average "low-cost" weekly budget for feeding a family of four was $155.

SECOND-GENERATION CRUSADER

Christine di Palma is a massage therapist in Hackettstown, New Jersey.

There was never a question about what Christine's daughter Marlie's diet would be like: It would mirror the fare her mom's own mother dished up.

"My mom was very holistic and way ahead of her time," di Palma says, recalling the then-fringy health foods such as wheat germ her mom served. "My mom had lost her father to heart disease when she was only 9 and was determined to protect her own family's health."

Today the di Palma family diet goes beyond organic. Gluten and sugar are generally off the menu—though, like any kid, Marlie does enjoy the occasional slice of birthday cake.

Marlie's propensity to inform fellow supermarket shoppers that, for example, their potato chips have artificial ingredients has made both mother and daughter the target of checkout-aisle eye rolling. And the fact that she's a slender child causes people to sometimes voice concern that she isn't getting enough to eat. (At 37 pounds, she is at a perfectly healthy weight for a girl her age and height.)

(continued on page 252)

GET THE INSIDE SCOOP

What mom doesn't give in to the calls of "We all scream for ice cream" every now and again? We found frozen treats that don't melt under scrutiny. The following cartons get our vote (with a cherry on top!). Here's our pint of view.

THE BEST NONDAIRY: So Delicious Dairy Free Vanilla Frozen Dessert

PORTION: ½ cup (2.8 ounces), calories 130, protein 1 gram, sugar 13 grams, fiber 3 grams, fat 3 grams

LIKE: This soy treat tastes just like the real deal, making it perfect for people who have lactose intolerance.

YIKES! Some dairy-free varieties—based on soy, coconut, and rice milk—can be high in fat and sugar.

THE BEST REDUCED CALORIE: Breyers French Chocolate Fat Free

PORTION: ½ cup (2.3 ounces), calories 90, protein 3 grams, sugar 13 grams, fiber 4 grams, fat 0 gram

LIKE: Our pick has less fat than many premium frozen desserts and also boasts fiber, which gives it more texture.

YIKES! Be cautious about fudge ribbons, which are mostly corn syrup with a dab of artificial dye.

THE BEST FROZEN YOGURT: Stonyfield Farm Organic Nonfat Frozen Yogurt

PORTION: ½ cup (3 ounces), calories 100, protein 4 grams, sugar 18 grams, fiber 1 gram, fat 0 gram

LIKE: This carton is packed with the good-for-your-gut bacteria that we love in yogurt.

YIKES! Other fro-yos lure you in by touting their "live and active cultures," but the actual yogurt portion can be minuscule.

THE BEST SORBET: Ciao Bella Blood Orange Sorbet

PORTION: ½ cup (3.6 ounces), calories 60, protein 0 gram, sugar 16 grams, fiber 0 gram, fat 0 gram

LIKE: A keeper! It's bursting with flavor, plus it has 50 percent of your daily vitamin C intake.

YIKES! Many sorbets have no real fruit in sight. Steer clear of ones with ice cream swirls, which drive up the calories and fat.

THE BEST ICE-CREAM SANDWICH: Julie's Organic Juliette Ice Cream Sandwiches

PORTION: 1 bar (1.4 ounces), calories 100, protein 2 grams, sugar 6 grams, fiber 0 gram, fat 5 grams

LIKE: You're less likely to overindulge because these organic novelty bars are portion controlled for you.

YIKES! Some ice-cream sandwiches swap the wafers for cookies, doubling the calories.

THE BEST ICE POP: Edy's All Natural Fruit Bars Strawberry

PORTION: 1 bar (3 ounces), calories 80, protein 0 gram, sugar 20 grams fiber 1 gram, fat 0 gram

LIKE: The real strawberry bits in this pop taste like summer. No high fructose corn syrup here.

YIKES! Beware varieties that resemble a chemistry project: Would you like a little sodium benzoate with your polysorbate 80?

ON THE MENU

Here's a sample menu at the di Palma home.

BREAKFAST: Gluten-free pancakes topped with sautéed apple slices and agave syrup, served with organic turkey sausage

LUNCH: Homemade hummus, olives, and lentil chips (which may be either brown-bagged for school or work or enjoyed at home)

DINNER: Tofu stir-fry with mixed vegetables and toasted sesame seeds

"It's hard when people tell me that Marlie is scrawny," says di Palma, who believes many parents are in denial about what is a normal size for a child.

"Once upon a time, pretty much all kids were skinny, and a heavy kid was really unusual. Now the reverse is true."

Di Palma believes that a diet free of chemical additives and very low in refined sugar and flour will help Marlie develop into the best student she can be. She is also confident that, as long as Marlie takes her dietary cues from her mom the way di Palma did herself, she'll avoid the health risks associated with obesity, including type 2 diabetes and heart disease.

THE HEALTHY CONVERT

Stacey Bogardus, 43, is a marketing manager in Indianapolis, Indiana.

In 2008, Bogardus faced big life changes. She was dealing with some nagging health issues, including gastroesophageal reflux disease (GERD), and she and her partner, Jami Sloan, were also about to start a family.

Both women grew up on standard American fare. By their mid-twenties, both thought they had improved their diets by eating more vegetables and opting for low-fat meats when they could.

"But we didn't even read labels," says Sloan. Organics weren't on the radar.

When Bogardus's GERD sent her to the doctor's office, he instructed her to take more antacids. That didn't work, so she turned to a naturopathic doctor who educated her about the value of choosing fewer processed and more organic foods. "Once you understand that many of the foods we think of as healthy are full of chemicals, you make different choices," Bogardus says.

For her, this realization hastened the end of buying conventionally raised meats and nonorganic produce. Sloan's pregnancy amplified the focus on nutrition, and by the time the couple's twins were born, their diet was approximately 75 percent organic. "It's not about being 100 percent organic," says Sloan. "It's about being 100 percent educated."

The boys do sometimes have fast food, especially if the family is traveling.

"But the kids don't go crazy for it like you would think. They actually kind of turn their noses up at fast food," says Bogardus. Like all kids, the twins favor familiar foods. For them, a homemade organic fruit smoothie is even better than a Dairy Queen milkshake.

It's more expensive, but spending a few extra dollars at the store is a small price to pay for better health, according to Bogardus, who's now off those antacids altogether and largely attributes this to improved eating habits. She also says that the boys have robust immune systems that easily fight off colds. But for Bogardus and Sloan, the real payoff will come when their sons grow up and make healthy choices for themselves.

"As parents, we have a responsibility to give them the best tools," says Sloan.

ON THE MENU

Here's a sample menu at the Bogardus-Sloan home.

BREAKFAST: Organic oatmeal with organic applesauce stirred in and milk

LUNCH: Organic Roll-Up (sliced organic turkey and cheese rolled up in a flattened slice of whole wheat bread) with soup and banana slices

DINNER: Organic chicken with couscous and green beans

CHAPTER 21

As Nature
Made Them

Genetically modified foods are all over your supermarket, but you'd never know it from the labels. How worried should you be?

Walk down the aisles of your local supermarket, and you'll find floor-to-ceiling shelves packed with food boasting nutritional benefits: whole grains in cereals, omega-3s in eggs, lycopene—that powerful antioxidant—in ketchup. But there are other ingredients hiding in these products, and most of us don't even know they're there. They're called genetically modified organisms (GMOs), and they're in 80 percent of the processed food on grocery store shelves—and a handful of whole foods as well, with perhaps more on the way soon.

A genetically modified food is one that has had lab-replicated genes from other plants, animals, and even viruses added to it in order to give it new characteristics—a resistance to insects, say, or to extreme heat and drought—that provide it an advantage in terms of hardy growth. Today, 91 percent of soy produced in the United States is genetically modified, as is 85 percent of corn and

88 percent of cottonseed, to name a few examples. Most GM crops are grown on large industrial farms and then processed into hundreds of other ingredients that show up in our food as corn syrup, soy lecithin, canola oil, cottonseed oil, or the sweeteners used in soups, spreads, and sauces—even infant formula. So ubiquitous have GMOs become, in fact, that unless a packaged food is certified organic or specifically labeled non–GMO, chances are it contains modified ingredients.

And it's not just processed foods. Hawaiian papaya, certain varieties of summer squash, and—as recently as December 2011—drought-resistant corn on the cob have also joined the list of crops that the Food and Drug Administration has reviewed for genetic modification in the United States. Pushing the envelope even further, the agency is now considering green-lighting genetically altered salmon, which would be bred with DNA that makes it grow to full size twice as fast as wild salmon.

HOW TO AVOID GM FOODS

Before any labeling changes can be made, you can protect yourself and your family. Here's how.

STAY AWAY FROM THE TOP EIGHT. The eight GM food crops are corn, soybeans, canola, cottonseed, sugar beets, Hawaiian papaya, and some zucchini and yellow squash.

GO ORGANIC. Certified organic food cannot intentionally include GM ingredients.

LOOK FOR THE "NON–GMO PROJECT" SEAL. This means the products have been independently tested and verified by the Non–GMO Project.

USE THE NON-GMO SHOPPING GUIDE. This easy-to-use online guide and completely free phone app takes the guesswork out of grocery shopping. Just go to nongmoshoppingguide.com.

SHOP WITH GM-FREE RETAILERS. Two large chains, Whole Foods Market and Trader Joe's, have banned GM ingredients from their house brands.

The controversy over GM food safety has swirled since the first altered foods were introduced in the early 1990s. Many scientists insist there's no proof that genetically modified food can harm human health. Their opponents counter that such claims cannot be responsibly made because there simply hasn't been enough research conducted—and there ought to be before consumers can buy them. Such arguments have persuaded 30 countries—including Japan, Australia, and the entire European Union—to ban or severely restrict GM crops. But the United States hasn't been persuaded.

In 1992, the FDA ruled that there's no "material" difference between genetically modified and traditional crops. In other words, if corn syrup made with genetically modified corn tastes, smells, and looks the same, has the same nutritional value, and can be used the same way as regular corn syrup, the FDA says that they are indeed the same.

"If we found that a genetically modified food was substantially different, we could require it to be labeled," says FDA spokeswoman Siobhan DeLancey. "But the way a food is produced doesn't make a material difference. We haven't found that GM foods as a class are different, or less safe, than conventionally processed foods."

Critics counter that the FDA's definition of a "material" difference is woefully behind the times.

"Right now, the FDA is doing 19th-century food labeling for 21st-century technology," says Andrew Kimbrell, an attorney and the executive director of the Center for Food Safety (CFS) in Washington, DC. "The idea that smell, taste, and feel are enough—that's something you do at a farmers' market. Not at a federal agency."

Many say what's needed is more and better peer-reviewed research. But no one is willing to fund it, says Marion Nestle, PhD, professor of nutrition at New York University in New York City and the author of *Safe Food*. A 2011 review of 94 articles in the journal *Food Policy* revealed that researchers who cast GMOs in a favorable light often had financial or professional conflicts of interest.

"The FDA and the US Department of Agriculture are essentially rendered powerless in the face of biotech lobbyists," Dr. Nestle says, "some of whom do stints as regulators themselves." Case in point: Michael R. Taylor, the FDA deputy commissioner for food, who oversees all of the agency's food and nutrition programs, was once vice president for public policy at Monsanto, a biotech company that produces an estimated 90 percent of the genetically modified seeds sold in the world. Monsanto's position is that "there is no need for or value in testing the safety of GM foods in humans."

"The burden [of proof] should fall on both the government and the companies that are producing these crops. It's their job to show it's safe," says Kimbrell of the CFS. "More than a decade ago, we predicted that genetically modified crops would cause environmental problems, and now it's happened. I suspect the same will be true for the human health risks."

Obligatory labeling that indicates the presence of GMOs by food manufacturers strikes many as a prudent first step. In 2011, a coalition including Physicians for Social Responsibility and the Ocean Conservancy launched the Just Label It campaign, asking the federal government to require labeling of GM foods. According to the organization, in early 2012, the 525+ partners of the Just Label It Campaign submitted a record-breaking 1.1 million comments to the FDA in favor of labeling genetically engineered foods. To date, the FDA has told them: "We haven't made a decision yet."

According to a 2010 Thomson Reuters poll, more than 90 percent of Americans think foods containing GMOs should be labeled. But for now, confusion abounds: Today, just 28 percent of Americans say they are aware that genetically modified foods are being sold in supermarkets, and of the shoppers who know, only about 1 percent guessed correctly that they were present in most processed foods. As a result, some food companies are going out of their way to assuage concerned consumers: "Non–GMO product verified" is one of the biggest trends in the natural products industry, with more than $1 billion in annual product sales.

"[Labeling] seems like a simple solution," says Maria Rodale, CEO and chairman of Rodale. "If given the choice, consumers might not choose to buy GM products. As of now, food manufacturers have decided not to give us a choice, which doesn't seem very American."

"Genetically modified foods offer consumers no advantage whatsoever," says Michael Pollan, author of *The Omnivore's Dilemma* and a pioneer of the sustainable food movement. "So far at least, these crops are no more nutritious, no tastier, and no cheaper than conventional. The real question is: Why would you eat this stuff?"

But in 2005, the World Health Organization announced that its opinion was that GM foods "are not likely, nor have been shown, to present risks for human health." Some animal studies suggest otherwise. This research has shown problems with reproductive, immune, and gastrointestinal systems, as well as organ damage and the possibility of accelerated aging. In one experiment at the University of Verona in Italy, a diet of GM soybeans damaged the liver cells in aging mice. Another revealed that ingesting genetically modified corn resulted in small changes to the rats' tissues, kidneys, and livers—though not enough to affect the animals' overall health.

In 2011, in one of the few human studies conducted so far, researchers at the University of Sherbrooke Hospital in Quebec tested the blood of 30 pregnant women and 39 nonpregnant women. They found traces of an insecticide present in the blood of 93 percent of the pregnant women and in 80 percent of umbilical cord blood. The most probable source, according to lead author Aziz Aris, PhD, is the genetically modified corn consumed as part of a normal diet in Canada, as it is in the United States. Dr. Aris wouldn't speculate about what health effects this might cause; that was beyond the scope of the study. But it was a shock to many, because GMO proponents have long claimed that GM proteins are destroyed during normal digestion. In every case, researchers have called for more tests and larger studies to help clarify risks.

"The scientific debate about the benefits and risks of these crops will continue for a very long time," says Gary Hirshberg, cofounder of the organic yogurt company Stonyfield, who is helping to spearhead the Just Label It campaign. "Without labeling, we're all involuntary participants in this giant experiment with our bodies—and our planet."

BUT WAIT, THERE'S MORE

Visit this site to add your name to the petition and learn more: http://justlabelit.org.

Part 5

MIND
MATTERS

CHAPTER 22

The Pursuit of Happiness

Do you believe you can feel better every single day—even in hard times? Dr. Andrew Weil says you can, but how will surprise you.

If you've ever wanted to be happier than you are, you're obviously not alone. But Andrew Weil, MD, the founder and director of the Arizona Center for Integrative Medicine at the University of Arizona in Tucson, is here to gently suggest that we might be going about it all wrong. Ever since he graduated from Harvard Medical School in 1968, Dr. Weil has been sounding the alarm about the wrongheadedness of the diagnose-and-drug model of health care. And now, with his new book, *Spontaneous Happiness*, he's fixing his gaze on what makes us truly happy, what to do when we're not, and how to better weather life's inevitable highs and lows. He says we can all feel better—much better—than we do.

There's an unspoken message in our society that we should all be happy all the time, and people are making themselves miserable trying to achieve it. Here's our interview with Dr. Weil, and his candid thoughts on the pursuit of happiness.

Dr. Weil: I don't think that happiness or depression is a mood we should be in all or even most of the time. Most of us look for happiness "out there," which renders it out of our control. The truth is, extremely negative and positive moods, like bliss and despondency, mark the edges of our emotional spectrum. They can help us discover a neutral midpoint of emotional health.

Prevention: And what is that midpoint exactly?

Dr. Weil: It's contentment, which is an internal state of well-being that's relatively impervious to life's transient ups and downs, and it's independent of what you have or don't have. If you hitch your moods to something external—getting a raise, a new car, a new lover—then what happens if that goes away? Contentment, on the other hand, is an inner feeling of calm; it's not dependent on external circumstances, possessions, or an episode of good fortune.

Prevention: So how do we foster contentment?

Dr. Weil: A good place to start is with a journal where you write down what

BREATHE EASY

We've all been told to "take a deep breath." Andrew Weil, MD, the founder and director of the Arizona Center for Integrative Medicine at the University of Arizona in Tucson, recommends we take that one step further with this exercise: "4-7-8 breath." "Doing this daily will induce a feeling of serenity," he says. "Over time, it'll give you greater emotional resilience—especially in hard moments."

1. Rest the tip of your tongue on the roof of your mouth, behind your top teeth.
2. Exhale completely through your mouth, with your lips slightly pursed, to make a whoosh sound.
3. Close your mouth and inhale deeply and slowly through your nose to a silent count of 4.
4. Keep your mouth closed and gently retain your breath for a silent count of 7.
5. Exhale slowly through your open mouth for a count of 8, making the same whoosh sound.
6. Repeat steps 3, 4, and 5 for a total of four breaths. Perform this twice daily for optimal results.

you're grateful for and then express thanks to key people in your life. Regularly practicing this sort of thinking is one of the best strategies for enhancing a sense of well-being. You should also try some form of meditation and deep breathing, which is free, and it's right under your nose! Breathing mindfully helps calm our nervous systems. It's an easy, powerful tool.

Prevention: But let's say you work two jobs, your parents are sick, your kids are struggling in school—how can you find time to do this?

Dr. Weil: I understand it's difficult, but breathing exercises literally take 5 minutes a day; sitting down quietly and meditating on your life takes just a few minutes too.

Prevention: So if we perform these exercises, how can we benefit, practically speaking, during hard times?

Dr. Weil: You may still experience a period of being thrown off balance, but you will be able to get through it more quickly, without becoming derailed. This kind of work, meditation especially, makes that possible: One of the primary benefits of meditation is it helps you find that calm center from which you can view the rest of your life without getting caught up in it.

Prevention: You also advance the notion that stress is actually a good thing. Why?

Dr. Weil: A stress-free life is a fantasy. Stress is not only inevitable but also useful. It keeps us in motion, keeps us changing. Obviously, if there is some external cause of stress that you can eliminate, you should, but it's much more important to learn techniques to protect your body and mind from the harmful effects of stress.

Prevention: What else can we do to sustain this kind of inner peace?

Dr. Weil: Spend time with people who have the qualities you want to emulate. We resonate with other people, so if you're around calm people, you become more calm yourself. There's a growing body of research that suggests contentment is contagious, as is depression.

Prevention: We'd like to know: What makes you content right now?

Dr. Weil: I spend hours every day in my garden, and I can see the results of it: It provides beauty; it gives me food; there is physical activity involved; I'm outdoors. That makes me happy.

CHAPTER 23

From Hectic to Happy

Love your weekends again with the following three key rules to get the stress out.

Come Friday, you're ready to relax and recharge, but too many of us sabotage our weekends by cramming in a month of chores or going zombie in front of the TV. Either way, the weekend is a bust. If you want to feel truly refreshed by Monday morning, take to heart the findings of a study showing that in addition to eating, relaxing, and sex, women enjoy themselves most when they're socializing, engaging in spiritual activities, and exercising. To make the most of your weekend, be sure to pencil in one activity from each category, and let the Rule of Three work for you.

RULE #1: USE YOUR SOCIAL NETWORK

Even if you cherish "just for me" time, organize at least one weekend endeavor where you can bring along a friend.

"Feeling connected and loved are among the biggest predictors of happiness," says Cassie Mogilner, PhD, assistant professor at the University of Pennsylvania's Wharton School in Philadelphia, who specializes in happiness research. Another bonus to socializing? It encourages us to spend our time and money on experiences, which research shows make us happier than material objects.

"When something is sitting on your shelf, you get used to it very fast," says Sonja Lyubomirsky, PhD, the author of *The How of Happiness*. So plan a Saturday-night outing to a play you've read about, or sign up for a cooking class with a pal. You'll enjoy the advantages for weeks or months to come.

Learn more about healthy friendships in "How Healthy Are Your Friendships?" on the opposite page.

POWER UP YOUR PLEASURE

Here are some more simple ways to get more "whew" into your weekends.

COMPRESS YOUR CHORES. To avoid having your to-do list take over, carve out 2- to 3-hour blocks for errands. "It allows you to say, 'There's a time for chores, and it's not that time,'" says Cassie Mogilner, PhD, assistant professor at the University of Pennsylvania's Wharton School in Philadelphia. Also consider whether there are things you can outsource—or ignore. Can you get your groceries delivered? And does the living room really need to be vacuumed once a week?

UNPLUG. After a week of making decisions, channel surfing can seem like just what the doctor ordered, but TV is less enjoyable than we think. Sociologists at the University of Maryland found that unhappy people watch 30 percent more TV than very happy people. Limit your Web surfing, too, since it comes with the added peril of checking work e-mail, which may invite stress into your time off.

RETHINK SUNDAY NIGHT. A new study says we remember unpleasant experiences as significantly worse if we expect them to recur, which might explain why so many of us ruin Sunday evening by dreading the week ahead. Instead, plan one of your Rule of Three activities for Sunday night: You'll fall asleep with a fond new memory, not a crash of nerves.

RULE #2: TRY SOUL FOOD

The more frequently that people attend religious services, the more content they are, according to a 2008 study in the *Journal of Economic Psychology*. Faith and prayer, regardless of religion, satisfy a basic need to feel part of something bigger than ourselves—and it turns out that volunteering can have a similar effect.

"People derive a lot of pleasure from helping others," continues Dr. Lyubomirsky. If prayer and volunteering aren't for you, try meditation or a restorative yoga class instead. New research shows that spiritual practices, such as regular mindfulness exercises, can actually change brain structure in a way that promotes a sense of well-being. So as a part of your Rule of Three this weekend, set aside some time for prayer or meditation, or volunteer to spend an hour or two at your local animal shelter. It'll lift your spirit—literally.

RULE #3: BREAK A SWEAT

"Exercise sparks the release of feel-good endorphins, but it also satisfies something more profound: the human need to perform and excel. Exercise helps you feel like the captain of your own ship," explains Dr. Lyubomirsky.

Although any fitness activity you enjoy is good, you'll enhance its benefits even more by taking it outdoors. A recent review of 11 studies that was published in *Environmental Science & Technology* found that people who exercised outside felt more energetic and were more inclined to keep at it. This is good news, because the rewards of physical activity are cumulative: The more you exercise, the clearer your mind. So as you arrange your weekend, schedule a trail walk, a bicycle ride, or a Sunday-night dance class with your partner. You'll close your weekend energized and ready to tackle the week.

QUIZ: HOW HEALTHY ARE YOUR FRIENDSHIPS?

You get more than just a little help from your friends, finds a new Brigham Young University study. You get good health, too, if you have the right ones. A strong social network, especially one with healthy pals, improves your chance of living longer by 50 percent. It doubles your odds of surviving cancer and wards off colds. Friends may even reduce your risk of cardiovascular disease, says lead study author Julianne Holt-Lunstad, PhD. And not having close bonds can be as bad for you as smoking up to 15 cigarettes a day.

Find out just how healthy your friendships are keeping you, and whether your group of pals is good for your mind and body.

Consider your group of friends as you take the quiz below. For each statement, answer "yes" or "no." Then add up the yeses to tally up how many of the following statements accurately describe your circle—and how many don't. Then look for the category that matches your score for assessment and advice.

On the whole, your pals . . .

_____ offer constructive help when you have a problem.

_____ don't insist on getting their own way in everything.

_____ haven't gained a lot of weight recently. (But even if just one has, count this as a no.)

_____ live close enough that you regularly meet face-to-face.

_____ rarely complain of being lonely or tell you they have no one to turn to but you.

_____ feel happy—either due to joyful events such as a son's wedding or finally buying a dream house—or just because.

_____ always listen with sympathy when you need to vent about work or a vexing family situation.

_____ feel free to ask you for small favors—such as picking them up at the airport or giving them free tax advice—and let you know your efforts are appreciated.

_____ don't act one way alone with you but differently in front of others.

_____ are not smokers. (If even one smokes, count this as a no.)

_____ might sometimes need your shoulder to cry on but are ready to return the favor.

_____ understand that you're human and can't always be perfect.

BEAT BLUE-MOOD MONDAYS

If you feel down in the dumps on Mondays, take heart: More than 75 percent of workers confess that Mondays make them so miserable, they don't crack a smile until after 11:00 a.m. They're also more likely to turn up late—and they complete less work. If this is your problem, ease into the day with some socializing.

"We're cavemen in city suits," says Alex Gardner, PhD, director at Insight Inquiry Research Consultancy in the United Kingdom, and we need to reconnect to our "tribe" to transition from weekend to work. So go ahead and gab: Your outlook—and your productivity—will be better.

_____ lose weight (if they need to) by eating right and/or exercising. (Even if only one friend has done this, count this as a yes.)

_____ try to be tactful and spare your feelings, even when they're telling you they disapprove of your choices.

_____ seem pleased with their relationships and/or family life.

_____ almost always answer your calls, show up, and make time for you.

_____ never stand you up, lie, or talk behind your back.

_____ have many other friends.

_____ chat back and forth with you (in person, by phone, or online) at least once a month.

_____ make you laugh out loud a lot.

Your Score

Add up the yeses and nos. Here's your score.

More yes than no answers: You have health-boosting buddies.

Your circle of friends makes you feel connected and needed. That's good news for your mood and your body.

"Supportive friendships can help you cope with stress, so you're less likely to suffer its negative physical and emotional effects," says Dr. Holt-Lunstad.

Better still, if a friend of yours—or even a friend of a friend—is happy in her life, chances are higher that you are (or soon will be) too, suggests a recent multi-university study. "Human beings are hardwired for emotional contagion," says study coauthor Nicholas Christakis, MD, PhD, professor at Harvard Medical School and Harvard University and coauthor of *Connected*. The caveat is that you must meet with your happy friend in person to "catch" her cheer: If she lives within half a mile of you, you're 42 percent more likely to be smiling yourself, but the effect decreases with distance.

While even far-off friends can bestow some health benefits, make sure that you have enough face time with closer chums to get the full effect. "Cell phones and social media are wonderful for enhancing relationships, but they're not a substitute," cautions Irene S. Levine, PhD, professor of psychiatry at New York University School of Medicine in New York City. "Plan time to see pals regularly—even if you have to multitask by meeting for a manicure or shopping. For long-distance loved ones, try to connect in person at least once a year."

About the same number of yeses and nos: There's room for improvement.

Your connections could use a checkup: Some of your pals may present problems for your well-being. If someone you're close to is often critical, competitive, needy, or untrustworthy, the relationship is unlikely to provide you with a stress-busting boost: Friends you feel ambivalent about raise your blood pressure (and potentially your risk of heart attack and stroke) even more than outright enemies, Dr. Holt-Lunstad found in another study series.

"People we just don't like are pretty predictable, so they're easier to cope with," she says. "Those toward whom we feel ambivalent, we care about on some level, so when they're unreliable or say something that hurts, it stings more."

3.5 THE NUMBER OF ACTUAL WORK HOURS PEOPLE COMPLETE ON MONDAYS

Just thinking about seeing someone with whom you have a love/hate relationship can up your anxiety level. And that kind of wary response means that when you share good news with these friends, you might disengage and not get the same uplift that sharing happy tidings would ordinarily give you.

Cutting these problematic pals out of your life often isn't necessary (or realistic), however. Instead, back off gradually and focus on cultivating ties with more straightforwardly supportive people.

More nos than yeses: Your circle's in need of treatment.

You might have landed in this category because while you do have pals, they're not exactly the picture of health themselves. Dr. Christakis's research shows that if you have a friend (nearby or far away) who becomes obese, you're 57 percent more likely to become obese too. Even a friend of a friend of a friend gaining weight can up the numbers on your scale, albeit to a lesser extent. Additional studies have found that the same is true of depression, heavy drinking, and smoking—apparently because we're heavily influenced by those around us.

But that doesn't mean you should drop a pal who's been stress-eating or unable to kick cigarettes. "Rather than focus on how your friends are adversely affecting you, concentrate on how you can affect them for the better," advises Dr. Christakis. Improving your habits will benefit you, and also your good example will send healthful ripples throughout your circle.

You might also have landed here because you have a loose collection of acquaintances but would describe few of them as close. Strengthening your social connections will serve you well, both physically and emotionally. People who feel lonely are less likely to get enough sleep, see the doctor when they need to, or handle everyday stress as well, according to a recent study conducted at the University of Arizona. That's why it's best to get back to making good friends—today.

CHAPTER 24

Serenity in a Sip?

Can you find bliss in a bottle? Is it possible to get calm from a can? We checked out the "chill out" claims of the new "relaxation" drinks. Here's what we discovered.

To unwind, perchance to sleep. . . . In our frazzled world, these seem to be elusive goals. Now manufacturers are trying to cash in on our need to relax, and the market is anything but sluggish. More than 350 varieties of so-called relaxation drinks have hit the shelves, with revenues expected to reach $73 million in a single year.

But do these relaxation beverages really work? Business is booming for these beverages, but they may be a bust. *Prevention* investigated and found some unpleasant surprises with these "serenity sips." Because they're not FDA regulated and many labels cite a proprietary blend, a buyer has no idea how much of each active ingredient—melatonin, valerian, L-theanine, and others—is actually captured in the can or bottle. There's also limited research on how these relaxants interact with one another. Nor are they all shelf stable: Some of these compounds degrade in liquid.

ON THE MELLOW MARKET

We sent five popular brands (two samples of each) to chemistry professor Joe Vinson, PhD, at the University of Scranton in Pennsylvania for analysis. He found that the amounts of active ingredients often differed from batch to batch. Even more shocking: In testing, some of the ingredients were barely present. Our advice? Save yourself the $3 (the average price per bottle).

Unwind with "Ultimate Relaxation": Our testing detected about half of the listed 3 milligrams of melatonin. (The hormone degrades up to 30 percent a month in liquids.) Even that much may be overdoing it.

Andrew Weil, MD, the founder and director of the Arizona Center for Integrative Medicine at the University of Arizona in Tucson, says that melatonin is a naturally occurring hormone that helps regulate your sleep cycle by sending the message to your brain that it's time for bed. He says that 0.25 to 0.3 milligrams might produce a more natural sleep cycle.

MiniChill, "Dr. formulated to make you feel calm, focused, and happy": The lab tests showed that this drink had only 0.7 milligram of L-theanine, nowhere near the 200 milligram dose that's proven effective. Instead, try gyokoru green tea for your L-theanine fix. This amino acid has been shown in studies to produce relaxing alpha waves in the brain.

TESTING THE WATERS

When you crave more zing than plain old H_2O can provide, there are now light and healthy options. These calorie-free herb- and fruit-infused waters refresh—without added sugar or preservatives.

HINT BLACKBERRY: The aroma of berries refreshes your senses, and the flavor is subtle.

METROMINT GOODBERRYMINT: You'll get a natural high from the cool scent and gentle hint of real mint.

AYALA'S HERBAL WATER GINGER LEMON PEEL: This organic water has a bold, spicy kick.

RelaxZen, "Promotes sleep, wake refreshed, reduce stress": This "sleepy" blend claims to include valerian, but we couldn't detect any of the active acid compound. That may be a good thing: Dr. Weil doesn't recommend taking it regularly, because it can cause dependency. Valerian root has been used throughout history as a sleep aid, but some research suggests that its ability to calm may be chalked up to a placebo effect.

Dream Water, "Drink to dream": This 2.5-ounce shot touts 5-HTP on the label. 5-HTP is an amino acid that spurs production of the brain's happiness chemical, serotonin. Unfortunately, this supplement breaks down easily in liquid, so it's not surprising we didn't detect any in our samples.

As for the neurotransmitter GABA, we found only 0.3 milligram in a serving—insufficient for any relaxing effects. GABA was shown to relieve anxiety in research published in 2006; however, the study was small, and further research is needed.

Mary Jane's Relaxing Soda, "Enjoy euphoric relaxation that's all natural, plain and simple": Kava, the only relaxant in this cola, is controversial: It's an herb that's been used as a ceremonial drink in the Pacific Islands for centuries because of its mellowing effect on mood. However, the FDA warns of potential liver damage from kava products. Dr. Weil recommends avoiding the herb in any form if you have liver problems, drink alcohol regularly, or just took acetaminophen (Tylenol).

CHAPTER 25

Energy Crisis Cures

This mother and daughter fought fatigue
at different times in their lives—and discovered
that a shared disorder was the cause.
Here's their story, in their own words.

Tired. Depressed. Lousy. That's how millions of women feel every day as they drag themselves out of bed and slog through life. According to the American Association of Clinical Endocrinologists, around 25 million people, mainly women, have thyroid disease. Half of them have no idea they have it. Here's one family's story.

THE DAUGHTER'S STORY

Heather McElrath, 39, says: "I had no idea what was wrong with me.

"I've always been really active. I hike, bike, and work out regularly at the gym. But a year ago, I started to feel totally burned-out. I blamed my crazy work schedule, plus the fact that I was training for my second triathlon. Two hours of swimming, biking, and running every weekend is tiring for anyone. But most active people aren't so wiped out that they can't lift their body off the couch afterward. I was. I'd go to sleep at 8:00 at night just to get through the next day. And I still felt foggy. I couldn't get motivated or make decisions. It was like someone turned the volume down on me.

"That wasn't the only problem. My immune system was also shot. Last winter, I caught every bug that was going around—colds, bronchitis, and a mild case of pneumonia (twice!). And while I wasn't gaining any weight, I wasn't losing it either, which was odd considering all the exercise I was getting.

"I thought a beach break would be the perfect fix, so in the spring, I went with four girlfriends to Tybee Island, Georgia. But I slept the whole time, and

A DOSE OF PREVENTION

Nothing will change your genetic risks, but at least you can avoid making them worse.

MAKE SURE YOU GET ENOUGH IODINE. This mineral is essential for the production of thyroid hormones. Years ago, before iodine was added to salt, flour, water, animal feed, and milk, iodine deficiency was rampant. Today, it's rare in America, though strict vegans can be at risk if they eliminate all eggs and dairy, as can the elderly if they avoid iodized salt to lower their blood pressure. Note: The salt in processed foods (the source of most sodium in our diets) is generally not iodine fortified. Take a multi that contains the mineral.

LIMIT SOY PRODUCTS. Soy isoflavones can suppress thyroid function if you eat too much. Menopausal women who take large amounts to ease symptoms are most at risk.

STEER CLEAR OF THYROID SUPPLEMENTS with seaweed extracts or the desiccated thyroids of pigs. They're sold over the counter, but they are unregulated, so you have no reliable way of knowing how much of the active ingredients you are actually taking.

BE SURE YOUR NECK IS COVERED WHEN YOU HAVE A MAMMOGRAM OR DENTAL X-RAYS. Although the risks are very slight, this low-dose radiation might contribute to thyroid cancer.

QUIT SMOKING. It doesn't cause hypothyroidism, but it can increase the severity and effects.

when we returned, I felt no better than when I'd left. I had to drop out of the triathlon.

"I knew my mom and grandmother had thyroid issues, so I began to wonder if this might be what was going on with me, even though my level of TSH (thyroid-stimulating hormone) had been normal a few months earlier when I'd seen my doctor for a checkup. I decided to get a second opinion, so I found a new internist. He ordered an additional blood test to check for Hashimoto's thyroiditis, an autoimmune disorder in which the immune system mistakenly creates antibodies that damage the thyroid gland. It's the leading cause of an underactive thyroid. This second test revealed that I had those thyroid autoantibodies.

"The doctor prescribed a low dose (0.25 microgram) of Synthroid, a synthetic version of thyroid hormone. I couldn't believe it, but by the very next day, I started to feel better! One pill in the morning every day, and I was back to being me. My brain was clear, and I started training again for another triathlon. This time, I intend to finish."

THE MOTHER'S STORY

Margaret McElrath, 63, says: "My story is much less dramatic than my daughter's.

"I was diagnosed with hypothyroidism when I was in my late twenties—about 10 years younger than Heather was when she received her diagnosis. I didn't have the same symptoms that she did—in fact, at the time, I didn't really notice that anything was wrong. I felt a little tired and a bit scattered, and I wasn't losing my pregnancy weight. But I was running around after a 3-year-old and working full-time! Who wouldn't be tired under the circumstances? I figured that was the way every working mom feels.

"So I was surprised when my doctor told me during a routine checkup that my thyroid was very enlarged. It's not like I could see anything was wrong. I didn't have a big bulge on my neck. I knew my mother had had some kind of thyroid problem, but since she never talked about her health issues—no one did back then—I forgot about it.

"Fortunately, my doctor realized immediately that having a thyroid gland so enlarged was abnormal, and he sent me to a specialist for an ultrasound. The technician gave me an oral dose of radioactive iodine, and the scan showed the same thing my internist had felt—that my thyroid was way bigger than it should be. The specialist explained that my body sensed I didn't have enough thyroid hormone, so it was working overtime in an attempt to produce more, and this was causing the gland to grow larger.

"My doctor put me on the same drug that Heather is taking, but a larger dose—175 micrograms. Honestly, I didn't think it was making a big difference in the way I felt until a few years ago, when my internist said it looked like I actually had too much thyroid hormone in my bloodstream. She lowered the dosage very slightly—and boy, did I feel it then. I was sluggish and lethargic. She put me back on my old dose, and I've been fine ever since."

DOCTORS SAY

Too little thyroid hormone leads to hypothyroidism, which is the most common form of thyroid disorder. It causes a slowdown in the body's metabolism, so you gain weight and feel sluggish, bloated, constipated, depressed, and forgetful. The most prevalent cause of hypothyroidism is an autoimmune disorder called Hashimoto's disease, though hypothyroidism can also be caused by inflammation of the thyroid, surgical removal of the gland, or even pregnancy. Undiagnosed, it can put you at risk of heart problems, infertility, and miscarriage. It's particularly dangerous in pregnant women during the first trimester, since it's been linked to developmental delays in infants, as well as lower IQ.

Too much thyroid hormone—known as hyperthyroidism—speeds everything up. Your heart races, and you feel anxious, irritable, or dizzy. You may also notice a too-rapid weight loss, difficulty sleeping, and, in some cases, a slight bulging of the eyes. The most common form of hyperthyroidism is Graves' disease, which is another autoimmune disorder.

It's not easy to diagnose thyroid disease. The thyroid is a small, butterfly-shaped gland that straddles the lower part of the windpipe in the front of the neck. This little gland produces powerful hormones, T3 and T4, that keep every system in your body running smoothly. When the hypothalamus senses that the level of thyroid hormone in your blood is low, it signals the pituitary gland to

DOCTOR'S ORDERS

Stephanie L. Lee, MD, PhD, director of the Thyroid Disease Center at Boston Medical Center and associate professor of medicine at Boston University School of Medicine, offers her advice.

Margaret and Heather are relatively fortunate: Their doctors recognized their thyroid disorders fairly early and took the right steps to treat them. According to the American Association of Clinical Endocrinologists, roughly 25 million people, mainly women, have thyroid disease. Half of them have no idea they have it; they just feel lousy. While the condition is most often diagnosed in those older than age 50, many patients have had symptoms that were missed or dismissed for years, even by doctors. That's because thyroid disorders develop slowly, mimic many other health conditions, and are often mistaken for the normal signs of stress or aging.

release thyroid-stimulating hormone (TSH) to kick-start production. Measuring your TSH is the gold standard for judging how well your thyroid is working.

But at what point is medication called for? That's a subject of debate. Until a few years ago, experts considered a TSH level of 0.5 to 5.0 normal. Anyone above that would be treated for hypothyroidism; below that, for hyperthyroidism. In general, doctors consider a TSH of 0.35 to 3.5 normal. But if your doctor is dismissing your symptoms, see another physician.

Fortunately, thyroid disease is easy to manage. For underactive thyroid, a daily dose of Synthroid is usually prescribed. For overactive thyroid, the regimen is more complicated and usually involves selectively destroying some of the thyroid tissue so that the gland doesn't produce as much hormone.

Because Synthroid is so effective at speeding up metabolism, some women with no thyroid problems clamor for it to help them lose weight or boost energy. Synthroid is not a weight loss drug and taking a medication you don't need can be risky. The fact that Margaret noticed a change when her dose was cut back shows just how delicate the balance of thyroid hormone in the body is.

CHAPTER 26

Earth Mothers
of Invention

*These six women launched successful organic
businesses. For them, every day is a labor of love.
Warning: Their passion is so contagious, you just
might want to change your own life next!*

Are you noticing more and more organic products popping up in the grocery
store these days? It's not your imagination: Organic foods—from soup to nuts—
are becoming more readily available.

According to the Organic Trade Association, the organic industry is growing worldwide. In the United States, sales of organic food and beverages grew
from $1 billion in 1990 to $26.7 billion in 2010. Organic food and beverage sales
represented approximately 4 percent of overall food and beverage sales in 2010.
Leading were organic fruits and vegetables, which now represent more than
11 percent of all U.S. fruit and vegetable sales.

The United States has one of the largest organic markets, along with Ger-
many and France. According to Organic Monitor estimates, global organic sales
reached $54.9 billion in 2009, up from $50.9 billion in 2008.

FIELD OF GREENS

Myra Goodman, 48, of Carmel Valley, California, cofounded (with her husband, Drew Goodman) Earthbound Farm.

Born and raised in New York City, Myra Goodman was headed for a career in international relations when she and her boyfriend (now her husband, Drew) stumbled upon the opportunity to run a small raspberry farm in California's Carmel Valley in 1984. The berries were being farmed conventionally at the time, and the owner gave Myra and Drew a 1-day tutorial on farm practices, including the application of pesticides. Call the couple naive, but until then, they had no idea how many toxic chemicals were routinely used in agriculture. The realization hit hard: "Oh my God, this food is grown with chemicals that you have to wear masks to handle, and it was going to be in our backyard!" says Myra, who was planning to live on the farm. The couple decided on the spot to farm organically. Never mind that they didn't know how. They bought *Rodale's Encyclopedia of Organic Gardening* and taught themselves.

Myra's experiment in country living might have ended as planned, after a year. But culinary changes were afoot in California, where Alice Waters, the formidable "mother of the organic movement," had started concocting delicious recipes with organic baby vegetables in her now-famous Berkeley restaurant, Chez Panisse. The Goodmans began supplying organic baby lettuces to local markets—then decided business was good enough to start shipping them nationwide under the label Earthbound Farm.

Today, an operation that started as 2.5 acres of raspberries has grown to 40,000 acres on 150 separate farms. It sells $475 million worth of produce a

A BETTER WAY TO MAKE YOUR BED

If you want to spoil yourself, splurge for some bamboo bedding. Bamboo feels silkier than even some sky-high-thread-count cotton sheets, it's hypoallergenic, and because it comes from an abundant plant, it's more sustainable. Look for 100 percent bamboo sets—not cotton blends—like the ones from BedVoyage ($99 to $169; amazon.com).

year, from arugula to zucchini, to 75 percent of the nation's grocery stores. And Myra has even blossomed into a cookbook author. But her proudest achievement is summed up in a single figure—14 million pounds. That's the amount of synthetic chemicals she and her workers spare the planet every year by farming organically.

DESIGNING WOMAN

Karen Stewart Brown, 41, of Ventura, California, cofounded (with her husband, Howard Brown) Stewart+Brown.

Early in her career, Karen Stewart Brown designed clothes for Urban Outfitters and J. Crew. But for all her knowledge of fashion, color, and fabric, she never fully understood the environmental impact of conventional cotton production. That changed after she took a job at Patagonia in 1998. She and her husband, Howard, considered themselves eco-conscious; they loved to hike and spend time in the mountains. But in 2001, Patagonia took employees on a tour of cotton fields in California's Central Valley.

"What I saw that day changed my life," she says.

As Karen describes it, the conventionally raised cotton was grown on acre upon acre of monocropped land that was devoid of wildlife, including birds.

"We weren't allowed to leave the bus, and you couldn't even go on the tour if you were pregnant because of all the toxic chemicals," she says.

By contrast, the next stop, an organic farm, was buzzing with life—sheep, goats, and children playing among the nearby fruit trees. It was like a Technicolor film after a black-and-white horror show. Karen vowed to herself, "I will pay double the price for a T-shirt if I know it's made with cotton from a farm like this." But would anyone else?

In 2002, Karen and Howard launched their own clothing line, Stewart+Brown, with tees and tops, dresses, and skirts made from fine organic cotton. In addition, they use linen and hemp fabric, because the flax and hemp plants are cultivated without the use of pesticides. And they import premium luxury cashmere from nomadic goat herders on the high plateau of Outer Mongolia. The USDA has no certification program for organic cashmere. But the nomads work as their ancestors have for generations—completely naturally.

"There's no need for pesticides because it's such an inhospitable climate—too high, too cold, too harsh," says Karen. There's nothing rough about her designs, though. Totally hip, Stewart+Brown shows that eco-fashion is about not just doing good—but looking and feeling good too.

SCENTS AND SENSIBILITY

Amanda Walker, 35, of New York City, founded A Perfume Organic.

As a child, Amanda Walker had a favorite game. She would play Avon Lady with her grandmother, filling a basket with her granny's beauty products, then ringing the doorbell for a pretend sales call. When she wasn't doing that, she would raid her mother's closet for lotions and perfumes—or mix her own scents from vanilla and almond extracts.

There was just one problem. Even as a child, Amanda couldn't tolerate many of the synthetic compounds in traditional perfumes, soaps, and shampoos.

"They would make me break out in hives or trigger my asthma," she says. "I thought it was just me." That was before she'd heard the words *multiple chemical sensitivities.*

In 2009, Amanda established A Perfume Organic. She distills scents from natural products such as pine needles, lemon balm, mint, and vanilla, then carefully combines the fragrance "notes"—top, middle, and bass—like a scented musical chord. Each bottle is hand-blended in her lab, which has USDA organic certification. Even better, some of her essential oils have antimicrobial properties, "so they calm your airways." A bonus: The recycled paper box is embedded with flower seed—so plant it and see what grows!

RECIPE FOR SUCCESS

Rachel Berliner, 58, of Petaluma, California, cofounded (with her husband, Andy Berliner) Amy's Kitchen.

Rachel and Andy Berliner were happily married and expecting their first child in 1987 when Rachel pulled a muscle in her leg. Unable to shop or prepare home-cooked dinners, she sent Andy to the local health-food store in search of frozen organic meals. All he could find was a bland lasagna.

HATS THAT LEND A HAND

Warm your head (and your heart) with a cap by Krochet Kids International, a nonprofit that sells winter wear made by women's cooperatives in Uganda and Peru. To find out more about the woman who knit your topper ($22 to $33), plug her name into krochetkids.org.

Rachel and Andy decided to start their own line of frozen foods that would be organic and flavorful too. Talk about a family affair. Rachel's mom contributed the first recipe—a vegetable and tofu potpie—and the couple named the company for their newborn daughter, Amy.

As the little girl grew, so did the business, Amy's Kitchen—along with the farms that Rachel and Andy now rely on to supply 100 million pounds of organic tomatoes, onions, and other veggies a year for 200 million lasagnas, pizzas, soups, and other meals. You can find the products anywhere from natural food stores to major chains.

"I love that Target carries them," says Rachel. "Part of my mission is to make organic food affordable."

And little Amy? Now 23 and a newly minted Stanford grad, she works in the company's small UK branch. And there's a second generation of customers too.

"I grew up on Amy's," moms write to Rachel. "Now I feed Amy's to my own kids."

LIFE IS A CABERNET

Barbara Shinn, 49, of Mattituck, New York, cofounded (with her husband, David Page) Shinn Estate Vineyards.

Barbara Shinn and her husband, David, were trendy New York restaurateurs in the 1990s. But as much as the couple enjoyed city life, they were drawn increasingly to the more gentle, holistic rhythms of a rural existence.

In 1998, they bought 20 acres of land on the North Fork of Long Island and decided to establish an organic vineyard and winery.

"We believed the earth needed to be saved by farmers," says Barbara. There was just one problem. "No one thought you could grow grapes organically on Long Island." The climate is too damp, fostering the growth of funguses that can easily destroy a crop. "That's why hotbeds of organic wine growing are places like the Napa Valley or Australia," she says.

But when Barbara and David stopped using chemicals, a surprising thing happened. They found that in a year of average rainfall, the crop was quite viable.

"The healthier the soil, the more the vines are able to withstand an onslaught of problems," she says. Funguses that form spores in soil, for example, are kept in check by naturally occurring microbes that also live in the ground—friendly microbes that most vintners kill off with chemicals. And by farming organically, they protect sensitive wetlands, bays, and estuaries from chemical-laced runoff.

Today, Barbara and David have a tasting room at their winery, where visitors can sample (and purchase) their estate merlot, cabernet, and sauvignon blanc. And they have renovated the 1880s house on the property as a B&B, called the Shinn Estate Farmhouse.

"We have only 20 acres, which is like a grain of sand on the face of the Earth," says Barbara. "But to have restored these 20 acres to their natural ecology is something I'm proud to have done. I only wish it could be 2,000."

FARMERS AT YOUR FINGERTIPS

Want an easy way to support local fare in your area? Try FarmPlate, a new site that takes the guesswork out of finding sustainable food near you. With more than 40,000 listings of farmers' markets, community-supported agriculture, restaurants, artisanal food and drink producers, and shops stocking organic fare, buying healthier eats is now no-excuses easy. Just type in your zip code at farmplate.com and chow down.

MY FAIR LADY

Tata Harper, 36, of Shoreham, Vermont, founded Tata Harper skin-care products.

Tata Harper lives on a pristine organic farm in Vermont, with her wildflowers. Her husband, Henry, raises organic grass-fed beef for local restaurants. It sounds like an idyllic existence. But it took a brush with death to jolt Tata and Henry out of their former fast-paced life in the Miami real estate world.

In 2002, at the age of 42, Tata's stepfather was diagnosed with an unusual cancer of the ureter. His youth and the cancer's rarity prompted his doctors at the Mayo Clinic in Jacksonville, Florida, to ask about his chemical exposures, suspecting a potential link with aniline dyes that are used in the textile industry. When that theory fell flat—Tata's stepfather is a veterinarian—they asked about his diet, his supplements, and even his shampoo, deodorant, and hand lotion.

"I found that really bizarre," says Tata. "What do beauty and grooming products have to do with cancer?"

No definitive link could be established. Still, the suggestion that troublesome ingredients might contribute to tumors, even if only rarely, was enough to prompt Tata to start shopping for natural beauty products. Most, however, contained only a smattering of natural ingredients—along with lots of chemicals. She decided to start her own, all-natural line.

It took 5 long years, during which she traveled the world and picked the brains of cosmetic chemists, herbalists, botanists, and even aromatherapists. In late 2009, she launched her eponymous skin-care line, Tata Harper—products from facial masks and cleansers to body oils that are 100 percent natural and mostly organic. Her Rebuilding Moisturizer, for example, contains rose water to hydrate the skin; essential oils of linden blossom, rose, bergamot, and geranium to nourish it; and raw honey from her farm to form a protective barrier. She concedes that her products are pricey but adds, "I feel that I'm contributing to people's long-term wellness." Not to mention happiness.

Part 6

BEAUTY
BREAKTHROUGHS

CHAPTER 27

The Defy-Your-Age Challenge

Are you doing things that make you look older than you are? Take this quiz to find out. Then follow the tips in the rest of Part 6 for our smart anti-aging advice, the best products, and more.

It's amusing to watch reality television contestants overhaul their images with cosmetic procedures, crash diets, and hair extensions. But even if you have the inclination—or the time and money—to make those changes, don't. Looking great for your age isn't about making other people think you have a good surgeon. It's about letting the vibrancy you feel on the inside radiate out—so much so that people actually notice. In essence, you want to defy your age.

"Defy is the perfect word; it implies taking an active role in caring for your appearance," says Vivian Diller, PhD, a New York City–based psychologist. "You're not throwing in the towel, but you're not going to extremes. It's a healthy, positive attitude."

The best place to start? Take our quiz.

WHAT'S AGING YOU? QUIZ

Grab a piece of paper and a pen. Read the statements below and make note of how many yeses you have in each category.

Improve Your Complexion Tone

- ☐ I wear sunscreen at the beach but not other times.
- ☐ I play DIY dermatologist all the time, squeezing blackheads and exfoliating my skin with scrubs.
- ☐ My skin color is uneven across my complexion. Some spots are redder, browner, or more mottled than others.
- ☐ I smoke or live with someone who does.

Smooth Your Skin Texture

- ☐ I am the queen of yo-yo dieting.
- ☐ I infrequently get eye exams.
- ☐ I don't usually wear sunglasses.
- ☐ An anti-aging, firming face cream seems like a better investment than sunscreen.

Get Younger-Looking Hair

- ☐ I fight my hair's natural texture when I style it, for example, straightening my curly hair or curling my straight hair.
- ☐ I like my hair to feel squeaky clean.
- ☐ I hardly ever get leafy greens, beans, or lean meats into my diet.
- ☐ I get my hair cut twice a year or less.

Better Your Body

■ When I stand naked in front of a mirror, it's easy for me to see which areas of my body have never been exposed to the sun.

■ I use body lotion only when my skin feels dry.

■ I do cardio exercise more often than strength-training.

■ I use anti-aging products on my face, but not anywhere below the chin.

YOUR RESULTS

Add up the number of Yeses you answered for each category. The category (or categories) with the highest numbers are the anti-aging goals you'll work on next.

Improve your complexion tone: see below.

Smooth your skin texture: see page 299.

Get younger-looking hair: see page 300.

Better your body: see page 301.

IMPROVE YOUR COMPLEXION TONE

It's easy to prevent redness, age spots, and pigmentation issues that add unwanted years. Here's how.

Be gentle. Avoid harsh scrubs and rough towel drying—and don't touch ingrown hairs or clogged pores. "Many women pick their skin, not realizing it can cause post-inflammatory pigmentation and scarring," says Heidi Waldorf, MD, a dermatologist at Mount Sinai Medical Center in New York City.

Stay away from smoke. "Cigarette chemicals get into your bloodstream and find their way to your skin, making it sallow and spotty," explains Alastair Carruthers, MD, a dermatologist in Vancouver. And avoid smoky rooms, because repeated exposure to smoke can also cause discoloration.

Say yes to daily SPF. You've heard it a million times, but have you gotten the message?

LOOK 10 YEARS YOUNGER

The following makeup moves will keep you looking rested and vibrant. Get ready to turn back the hands of time! Have firmer, smoother-looking skin with the wave of a makeup brush. We like to call it "fake-it makeup."

HAVE A FAUX-TOX. Soften brow lines by blending a foundation slightly lighter than your usual shade over the center of your forehead; it creates a highlight that blurs the look of wrinkles. Finish with Sonia Kashuk Brightening Powder ($10; Target).

LIFT YOUR BROWS. High, full brows look youthful and help define all your features, says Los Angeles makeup artist Brett Freedman. Use a brow powder or pencil a shade lighter than your hair color to fill in sparse areas, and then sweep a fine line right above the top of the arch. Try Wet n Wild Eyebrow/Eyeliner Pencil ($1; drugstores).

CAMOUFLAGE CROW'S FEET. Nix heavy cover-up, which makes lines more obvious, says Matin Maulawizada of Laura Mercier Cosmetics. Instead, brighten the area with concealer under the outer third of your lower lashes and a creamy highlighter such as Benefit Ooh La Lift ($22; benefitcosmetics.com) just below any lines.

REDUCE "PARENTHESES." To diminish the lines that run from your nose to your mouth, apply concealer one shade lighter than your skin over the shadow below the fold only, not over the entire crease, says Maulawizada. This pro trick reduces the appearance of a defined edge. Try Laura Mercier Secret Camouflage ($30; lauramercier.com).

PEP UP YOUR POUT. "The sides of the mouth tend to droop with age," says Joanna Schlip, makeup artist for Physicians Formula. "To lessen the effect, brush highlighter on the corners and concealer just below the outer edges of your lower lip to minimize shadows." Try Sonia Kashuk Multi-Purpose Nylon Brush ($6; Target).

GET A SURREAL PEEL. Mimic the results of a chemical peel—smooth, glowing skin—by applying a line-filling, anti-aging primer before the rest of your makeup. Try RoC Brilliance Anti-Aging Face Primer ($24; drugstores).

HAVE A LIGHT LIFT. To give your whole face a visual lift, use bright blush on your cheeks, then dab a flesh-toned illuminator just above the blush. Try Philosophy Divine Illumination Love at First Light Ageless Skin Luminizer ($33; philosophy.com).

"Even if you don't sunbathe, you can get freckles and broken capillaries simply from walking to the car each day without sunscreen," says Dr. Carruthers.

Use illuminating makeup. With age, melanin production decreases, which means even the healthiest, most even complexion lacks the flush of youth, according to makeup artist Laura Geller. Balance out your skin with a foundation that has brightening ingredients built in, such as Revlon Age Defying with DNA Advantage Cream Makeup ($15; drugstores).

Don't go to extremes. Jet black and platinum blonde are notoriously hard-to-pull-off hair-color hues. That's because they contrast too much with skin tones and can make your complexion look dull or draw attention to redness or imperfections, says Michael Canale of the Canale Salon in Beverly Hills, California.

Be cheeky. Dust on a bronzy-pink blush for added radiance. "On mature skin, it's more flattering than a poppy pink or mauve," Geller explains. Try Laura Geller Blush-N-Brighten with Brush in Pink Grapefruit ($35; qvc.com).

SMOOTH YOUR SKIN TEXTURE

Saggy skin, wrinkles, and rough patches add digits to your perceived age. Here's how to stay firm and unlined.

Slip on shades. "Large lenses help protect the skin around your eyes from sun damage and prevent you from squinting, which can worsen wrinkles," says Ranella Hirsch, MD, a dermatologist in Boston. Get your eyes examined too. Squinting as you try to focus can also deepen lines.

Maintain your weight. If the choice is between constantly losing and gaining, or settling for a few extra pounds, do the latter. "As we age, the dieting cycle leads to an unfirm complexion because skin can't bounce back as easily," says Dr. Waldorf.

Stock up on sunscreen. It's easy to make a connection between sunlight and sun spots, but rays can also weaken skin's supportive structure, making it crepey and causing roughness. As Dr. Hirsch points out, there's no reason to spend lots of money trying to firm up your complexion later when you can spend a little on sunblock now.

Firm your face. The anti-agers you've been using reduce lines and roughness, but why not take your texture improvement one step further with a foundation that doubles as a lifting treatment? L'Oreal Paris Visible Lift Smooth Absolute Foundation ($16; drugstores) contains collagen-boosting retinol and hydrolyzed elastin to plump skin with moisture. For the best results, apply it in natural light.

"The biggest mistake that women make as they get older is trying to put on makeup in front of a tiny mirror in a poorly lit bathroom," Geller says.

Open your eyes. Apply a matte taupe or soft brown shadow from the lash line almost to the brow, then use an angled shadow brush to apply a slightly darker shade just above your lid crease. "Most women put the darker shade in the crease, but a bit higher detracts from sagginess better," says Geller.

Adjust the tone of your hair color. "Hues that complement your skin's natural undertones look more youthful," Canale says. Warm undertones? Try golden blondes or caramel-tinged browns. Wheat-hued blondes or ash browns are better for cool undertones.

GET YOUNGER-LOOKING HAIR

Start improving the health of your hair and scalp now to take time off your strands—and years off your looks.

Eat iron-rich foods. "I've done blood work on thousands of women with thinning hair, and I rarely discover medical issues; more frequently, I discover low iron levels," Dr. Carruthers says. An iron-rich diet can't grow back hair lost due to genetic causes, but it can maintain thicker, more youthful-looking strands.

Embrace your texture. Healthy curls are younger than starched-straight strands, while shiny, straight locks look better than plasticky curls. Moral of the story: A low-maintenance 'do means no hot-tool damage.

Wash less and cut more. Shampoo (even good stuff) dries your hair, so limit yourself to three washes a week. And get a trim every 6 to 8 weeks to remove the dull, dry tips that really age you. "No product can make the ends as healthy as new hair growing in," says Dr. Carruthers.

Soften your style. Spiky haircuts or blunt tips that go against the natural contours of your face can create harsh shadows that call attention to wrinkles. Ask for layers that frame your face, adding a pretty softness, suggests Roxy Coberly of Woodley & Bunny Salon in Brooklyn.

Thicken up. Give straight or wavy hair a volume boost with the right blow-drying technique: Use a paddle or round brush to pull the hair on your crown toward the ceiling as you dry it. Choose a dryer with a concentrator nozzle, which focuses airflow to reduce frizz.

Add shine from the inside out. For glossy hair—a hallmark of youth—repair your strands so the cuticle layer lies smoothly and reflects more light. An oil-based serum, such as Ojon Damage Reverse Instant Restorative Hair Serum ($25; ojon.com), penetrates to help fix damage.

BETTER YOUR BODY

A spotted chest, wrinkly hands, and rough, dry arms and legs are true-age give-aways. Get back your youth with these fixes.

Cool off. "Every dermatologist would agree that dry skin can make you look older," says Dr. Hirsch. Moisturizing helps, but there's an even easier fix: Take shorter, cooler baths and showers, because hot water dehydrates skin.

Lift weights and dig in. Aerobic exercise is good, but strength-training is better if saggy skin on your body is the issue. "Skin looks more taut over supportive muscles," Dr. Hirsch says. If you're hungry postworkout, eat! "After a certain age, a few extra pounds can actually help your face look younger," she says.

Do more naked. Smooth on lotion or sunscreen after you dress, and you might miss areas. Instead, apply products straight out of the shower so you remember to extend application to your neck, chest, and hands too.

Maximize your manicure. A pop of color draws attention to your nails—away from any spots or wrinkles. Go for red or bright pink, and avoid supertrendy hues; they make it seem like you're trying too hard to look younger.

Prime your skin. Smooth a face primer like Maybelline New York Instant Age Rewind Primer Skin Transformer ($10; drugstores) on your neck and chest.

THE AGE ERASERS

Getting older might be inevitable, but how you look as you age is controllable. "Genetics predetermines only about 20 percent of how your looks change over the years," says Dr. Waldorf. "The rest is affected by daily habits, your lifestyle, and the products you use." That's where *Prevention* steps in: We're unveiling 10 anti-aging products scientifically proven to change your skin, body, and hair for the better.

Prevention reviewed more than 900 products launched between April 2010 and April 2011 and selected 61 finalists. The shampoos and conditioners were then blind-tested at TRI/Princeton, an independent lab; the hair treatments were tested on 5 to 10 women over the course of 4 weeks under the supervision of a cosmetic chemist. The face and body products were used by 5 to 10 women for 6 weeks, and our dermatologist judges determined the winners by analyzing testers' skin before and after, reviewing their written evaluations, and using complexion analysis machines, such as the Visia Complexion Analyzer by Canfield, to calculate changes in the number of wrinkles and spots.

How do you know which of the 10 winners is right for you? Find the anti-aging goal(s) you identified in the quiz on page 296, and then look for the products identified as being beneficial for those goals.

THE BEST DAY MOISTURIZER

L'Oreal Paris Youth Code Day Lotion SPF 30 ($25; drugstores)

Improve your complexion tone.

Smooth your skin texture.

With sunscreen, hydrating ingredients, and peptides that boost collagen production, this lotion is the ultimate multitasker. Women who used it had more vibrant complexions after 6 weeks and saw bigger decreases in the number of spots and wrinkles than those testing other products, according to judge Tina Alster, MD, clinical professor at Georgetown University. The lotion also prevents future damage with adenosine, which fuels healthy cell function, and biolysat, a good bacteria that helps skin fight off environmental damage.

THE BEST NIGHT TREATMENT

Origins Plantscription Anti-Aging Serum ($55; origins.com)

Improve your complexion tone.

Smooth your skin texture.

Some anti-agers are irritating, but this serum won with a gentle combo of collagen-stimulating botanicals and an extract from the West African Anogeissus tree that boosts production of fibrillin, a glycoprotein "that makes skin elastic and springy," according to judge David J. Goldberg, MD, clinical professor at Mount Sinai School of Medicine in New York City. Testers using it saw up to a 30 percent improvement in the number of fine lines they had—results that rival using a prescription anti-ager for a similar time period.

THE BEST EXFOLIATING TREATMENT

Clarins Bright Plus HP Gentle Renewing Brightening Peel ($38; clarins.com)

Improve your complexion tone.

Smooth your skin texture.

This goes on like a toner but does the job of a scrub, dissolving dead skin cells with glycolic and salicylic acids for a smoother, more even-toned complexion. On average, testers who used it saw a 33 percent improvement in texture and a reduction in pore visibility. Judge Dr. Waldorf says the peel works best used before an anti-aging moisturizer or treatment because "it boosts other products' effectiveness by allowing them to penetrate deeper."

THE BEST EYE CREAM

Dr. LeWinn by Kinerase Lift & Resculpt Anti-Wrinkle Eye Cream ($28; Walgreens)

Improve your complexion tone.

Smooth your skin texture.

Featuring dill extract—an antioxidant that reduces wrinkles, according to a study in the *International Journal of Cosmetic Science*—this cream decreased the length and depth of lines around testers' eyes up to 40 percent and, in some cases, reduced spots and redness. The peptide-rich formula also stimulates collagen production, "which can improve the look of dark circles," according to judge Marina Peredo, MD, associate clinical professor at Mount Sinai School of Medicine in New York City.

THE BEST NECK CREAM

Elizabeth Arden Ceramide Plump Perfect Ultra All Night Repair Moisture Cream for Face and Throat ($66; elizabetharden.com)

Better your body.

Many women neglect the skin below their chins, a difficult area to treat, but testers using this cream found it is possible to make a difference. The peptides, ceramides, and hibiscus extract helped plump fine lines and slightly reduce their appearance. Dr. Hirsch also liked that it has "vitamins C and E, which can protect against free-radical damage and hyper-pigmentation."

THE BEST HAND CREAM

Avon Anew Clinical Luminosity Pro Brightening Hand Cream SPF 15 ($15; avon.com)

Better your body.

Give signs of aging the one-two punch with this cream's combo of retinol and glycolic acid, which softens lines and fades discoloration. Testers loved how it improved the look of thin, crepey skin and even lightened age spots in some cases.

"I used to tell patients they could only get these benefits from laser treatments," says judge Alastair Carruthers, MD, clinical professor at the University of British Columbia.

THE BEST LIP TREATMENT

Blistex Five Star Lip Protection SPF 30 ($2; drugstores)

Smooth your skin texture.

This balm smooths lips and moisturizes with calendula extract, glycerin, and safflower and coconut oils to reduce the appearance of fine lines. Testers gave the "nongreasy," "hydrating" formula better ratings than other products in the category—including a $38 lip plumper!—but a key reason it scored the top spot was its high SPF level, says judge Mary Lupo, MD, clinical professor at Tulane University School of Medicine in New Orleans.

THE BEST SPOT FADER

Specific Beauty Skin Brightening Serum ($30; specificbeauty.com)

Improve your complexion tone.

Ever wish you could take an eraser to your brown spots? Now you can: This paraben- and fragrance-free serum has "a killer combo of retinol and licorice extract that faded brown spots, as well as anti-inflammatory gingerroot extract and niacinamide, which prevents new flecks," according to judge David Bank, MD, assistant professor at Columbia University/Presbyterian Hospital in New York City. On average, testers had 25 percent fewer brown spots after using it—and one tester had 50 percent fewer (results that will last if they're vigilant about wearing sunscreen).

THE BEST BODY MOISTURIZER

Super by Dr. Nicholas Perricone Superhero Body Sculpting Serum ($35; sephora.com)

Better your body.

This lotion, which works well under sunscreen, packs anti-agers once found only in face products, such as polyphenols to protect against environmental damage and glycolic acid, which helps smooth rough patches. Dr. Carruthers noticed it faded spots on several testers' arms, and almost all of the testers commented on the lotion's skin-firming effect, a benefit of the caffeine, which decreases water content in fat cells beneath the skin.

THE BEST HAIR TREATMENT

Redken Time Reset Corrective Defense ($20; redken.com for salons)

Get younger-looking hair.

This leave-in lotion features "a rare, superlight silicone that forms an undetectable web around strands to make them more full and shiny, while protecting against breakage and split ends," according to judge Ni'Kita Wilson, cosmetic chemist and vice president of research and innovation at Englewood Lab in Englewood, New Jersey. Testers said the "weightless formula" left their hair "softer and more manageable."

CHAPTER 28

The Hair of Your Dreams

You can have a good hair day, every day, with the following terrific tips and top products.

Bad hair days might be the stuff of sitcoms, but are they really a big deal? You bet. One study in Canada found that worldwide, one in four women has passed on a social event, one in five has shunned physical activity, and others have avoided joining a club (18 percent), going to a job interview (16 percent), or hitting the beach, spa, or swimming pool (29 percent) because they experienced discomfort with their looks. And certainly a big part of how we feel about how we look is wrapped up in our hair.

Hair changes are probably one of the most obvious signs of aging. Two major challenges many women face are thinning hair and graying hair. But you can fight—or at least work with—both. Here's how.

BULK UP THINNING HAIR

Many women discover that their hair is not as thick and full as it once was. Try these treatments and styling ideas to fight back.

Roxy Finn, 47, first noticed her hair was thinning in her twenties, but it's gotten worse in the past few years.

"It's one of the most devastating things I've ever had to face," she says. "Women are supposed to have thick, sexy hair, so it's a big chunk of your sexiness down the drain—literally!"

Initially, Finn thought the thinning might have been due to perming her hair, but after consulting her primary care doctor, gynecologist, and dermatologist, she learned that the real problem is a genetic predisposition. Put simply, her hair is no longer growing in as thick or as long as it did when she was younger.

Finn is not alone, as 50 percent of women experience some kind of hair loss by age 50.

"It's far more common than people realize," says Robert Leonard, DO, founder of Leonard Hair Transplant Associates in Cranston, Rhode Island. But even though the problem is widespread, it's only now that help is more readily available.

"More women in my practice are addressing this condition," says Mary Gail Mercurio, MD, associate professor of dermatology and obstetrics and gynecology at the University of Rochester in New York. "That's encouraging, because the sooner hair loss is diagnosed, the better the chances of finding its cause and successfully treating it."

The Root Cause

"We all shed around 100 to 150 hairs per day," says Paradi Mirmirani, MD, a dermatologist in Vallejo, California, who specializes in hair disorders. But if you're losing more than that (you can tell if you see clumps of hair in the shower drain), your part is getting wider, or your hair has become significantly finer, you may be dealing with female pattern hair loss, which is a genetic condition that affects 30 million American women. Although FPHL (which is also called androgenetic alopecia) can begin as early as your twenties, it's most common after menopause.

"Multiple genes play a role, and they have an equal probability of being inherited from your mother's or father's side," explains Dr. Mercurio.

Although this type of hair loss doesn't necessarily indicate a medical issue, you should consult your doctor to rule out a thyroid problem, iron deficiency anemia, or an excessive level of male hormones (common when you have polycystic ovarian syndrome or when estrogen levels drop off around menopause). These conditions might cause a different type of hair loss or aggravate FPHL if left untreated.

If your doctor determines that you don't have these other, more serious health issues, or resolving them doesn't minimize symptoms, your next stop is the dermatologist's office. She will perform a scalp exam and take a detailed medical and family history to determine why your hair is thinning and help you develop a treatment plan.

BODY BUILDERS

You can choose from hundreds of products that promise to pump up thinning hair. So we did the research for you, sending the latest shampoos, conditioners, and stylers to *Prevention* readers to test. Check out their favorites here.

UMBERTO BEVERLY HILLS VOLUME SHAMPOO: ($9; Target) Our tester said this shampoo with hydrolized silk proteins left hair "full of body" and was helpful plumping strands "on the top of my head."

FULL BY LIVING PROOF ROOT LIFTING SPRAY: ($26; livingproof.com) "I use this every day," said a tester of this spray with an MIT-developed polymer. "It makes hair look fuller and thicker."

JOICO CLINICURE LIFTING FOAM VOLUMIZER: ($14; joico.com) Formulated with botanical extracts, this foam gives "extra lift on the crown area" while "controlling frizz."

OJON VOLUMIZING 2-MINUTE HAIR MASK: ($30; ojon.com) This whipped treatment "conditioned without weighing hair down" and "made combing easier," which "helped to prevent breakage."

Natural Healing

Although you can't change your genes, you can do some things to protect the hair you have. But think lifestyle changes—not hope in a jar.

Change your diet. If you're vegetarian or anemic, you might lack adequate iron, which is essential for strong, healthy hair. Make sure you're eating plenty of leafy greens—such as spinach, kale, and chard—and beans, tofu, or lean cuts of red meat, which are all great sources of iron as well as biotin and zinc, two nutrients that might also play a role in hair growth.

Massage your scalp. Many pros suggest scalp massage for clients with thinning hair. "Use your fingertips and a bit of argan or coconut oil to rub in a circular motion for several minutes before you shampoo," says John Masters, owner of John Masters Organics Salon. Mary Lupo, MD, clinical professor of dermatology at Tulane Medical School in New Orleans and a *Prevention* medical advisory board member, says the theory is that massage temporarily increases circulation to the scalp, which might pump hair follicles with the nutrients needed for hair growth.

Doctors' Orders

Following a holistic approach that incorporates diet tweaks and other alternative therapies might thicken hair, but some women still need medical help to see significant regrowth.

Try an OTC cure. Currently, the best (and only FDA-approved) treatment for hair loss—no matter what its cause—is topical minoxidil, the drug used in

FIX YOUR FRIZZ

John Frieda Full Repair Touch-Up FlyAway Tamer ($10; drugstores), a new gel applied with a mascara-like wand, claims to control wispies that pop up along your hairline or escape from buns or ponytails in humid weather. Our testers said it was more effective than hair spray for locking down wayward strands; they also liked how it didn't make hair crunchy or sticky.

REVIVE THOSE ROOTS!

Want to sap greasy roots and add volume to your hair? Dry shampoo could be your new mane squeeze. But before you buy one, try a smart substitute from your kitchen: cornstarch.

Sprinkle a pinch along your part, tousle your hair to distribute throughout, then brush or style as usual.

Rogaine, which is an OTC treatment available in mousse or liquid formulas. "It's not clear exactly how minoxidil works, but studies show it lengthens the growth phase of your hair," says Dr. Leonard. Applying 2 percent minoxidil to the scalp twice daily has been shown to produce minimal regrowth in 40 percent of women and moderate regrowth in 19 percent. Possible side effects include itching and redness of the scalp.

Consider a prescription remedy. If you don't respond to minoxidil, your doctor might prescribe antiandrogen medications, which might slow hair loss and even stimulate growth in some women. "They inhibit male hormones that can exacerbate hair loss," explains Dr. Mirmirani. In select cases, she may prescribe finasteride, a 5-alpha reductase inhibitor, which blocks an enzyme that regulates the production of androgens. Because the medication causes birth defects, it is FDA approved only for men. "In premenopausal women who are no longer childbearing, finasteride can be used off label," Dr. Mirmirani notes.

Style Smarts

Don't underestimate the importance of the right cut, color, and styling routine.

Switch your part. "Changing the direction of your part can really help thinning hair," says Nexxus Creative Director Kevin Mancuso. Hair tends to lie flatter against the scalp when brushed repeatedly in the same direction. If you typically part your hair on the left, flip it to the right, so it's more likely to stand away from your scalp and look more voluminous.

Prevention.com asked 1,371 women ages 18 to 65 (mean age: 50) what they thought about their hair hue.

Seventy-two percent of women with gray hair dye it. Here's why:

- 51 percent think they would look older if they stopped dyeing.
- 18 percent have dyed so long, they're not ready to find out what's underneath.
- 14 percent don't feel like dealing with the growing-out process.
- 10 percent think having gray hair would impact them negatively at work.

Twenty-eight percent of gray-haired women don't dye. Here's why:

- 40 percent like their natural hair color as is.
- 23 percent are worried about chemicals in the dye.
- 21 percent say it costs too much to dye on a regular basis.
- 16 percent say they'd feel like they were trying to be someone they're not.

Keep cool. In general, the less heat you use, the better. "Styling with heat can damage the hair shaft," says Dr. Mirmirani. Air-dry whenever possible, and if you must use heated tools, pick those with adjustable settings and keep them on the lowest level. "This won't affect hair growth, but you'll see less of the breakage that makes hair look even thinner," Dr. Mirmirani says.

Brush with care. Used in conjunction with a blow-dryer, round metal brushes can heat up significantly, and some brushes with hard plastic or metal bristles can cause breakage, according to Angelo David, owner and creative director of New York City's Angelo David Salon. Instead, try a brush made of gentle boar bristles or flexible nylon.

Get a volumizing cut. In most cases, shorter cuts are kinder to thinning hair. "The longer your hair grows, the more likely it is that sections will separate and reveal your scalp," explains Mancuso. Whatever length you choose, ask for interior layers, which are placed throughout your cut, not just on the ends, to add fullness.

Color strategically. Bleaching or significantly lightening your hair color all over can cause damage or breakage, but well-placed highlights hide thinning by making your hair color more similar to the color of your scalp. Plus, the dye expands the hair shaft slightly so it appears thicker, according to David.

SEIZE THE GRAY

Getting gray, white, or silver hair is a natural part of aging. But no one said we have to *like* it. Around half of American women over age 25 color their hair.

The Root Cause

"The process of going gray—which occurs as follicles stop producing melanin— is determined by DNA, not diet or other factors," says David Bank, MD, director of the Center for Dermatology, Cosmetic and Laser Surgery in Mount Kisco, New York.

Although new research on mice shows that exercise might stave off the loss of hair pigment, while stress may speed up the process, these findings haven't

THE GRAY ALL-STARS

Who says gray can't be great? Here are some celebs sporting gray.

- Singer Emmylou Harris
- Model Nicky K
- Makeup artist and model Cindy Joseph
- Former congresswoman Jane Harman
- Actress Jamie Lee Curtis
- Actress Helen Mirren
- Meryl Streep as Miranda Priestly in *The Devil Wears Prada*
- Novelist Louise Penny
- Essie Weingarten, the founder of Essie Cosmetics

been replicated in humans. So even though it seems as if every president goes gray after a few months in office, there's no proof (yet) that stress is the cause.

Even the seemingly accelerated speed at which certain sections go gray (temples first for some, the crown area for others) and the exact shade of gray you get (white, charcoal, or any of the other variations) are genetically predetermined.

"Your head has roughly 100,000 hair follicles, and each functions autonomously," Dr. Bank explains. "If one runs out of melanin, even if you pluck the resulting gray hair, there will be no impact on surrounding follicles—nor is your lifestyle likely to affect the color."

"YOU LOOK GREAT IN GRAY"

That's what people will say if you accent your hair with the right clothes and makeup.

"When you see a really attractive gray-haired woman, she's often wearing charcoal and silver clothing, which makes her gray hair even more striking," says a colorist at the Rossano Ferretti Hairspa in New York City. You don't need to restrict your wardrobe to that color family, but black, white, shades of gray, and jewel tones (ruby red, sapphire blue, and deep purples) are your best bets. Avoid earth tones such as beige and olive, which can wash you out.

If you're going to commit to gray, the labor you save coloring your hair should be switched to putting on makeup, since gray hair tends to make your complexion appear dull. The best place to start? Blush. "Go for shades like apricot, peach, and rose—not beigy or tawny colors," suggests Yvette Gonzalez, senior stylist and makeup artist at Sahag Workshop in New York City. "They make your skin tone look muddy next to gray hair."

Most important of all: Groom your brows. Trim wayward hairs (grays tend to be wiry), and define your arches with a taupe pencil so they don't disappear.

DO THIS AND DYE LESS!

You can save your color—and your hard-earned cash—with the following tricks that cut down your dye sessions each year. (Read: less time soaking up chemicals.) Your hair—and scalp!—will thank you.

STEP 1: PICK A DO-MORE DYE. Clairol Natural Instincts at-home hair-coloring kits ($9; drugstores) feature a new Week 2 ColorFresh Refresher. Applied 14 days after dyeing, this pack deposits color-enhancing molecules that renew your shade in 5 minutes.

STEP 2: WASH THIS WAY. Use shampoo with polyDADMAC, a liquid crystal proven in the *International Journal of Cosmetic Science* to rebuild hair's protective layer so color is locked in longer. Find it in the Pantene Pro-V Color Hair Solutions line (from $4; drugstores).

STEP 3: GIVE IT A GLAZE. Three weeks after dyeing, apply a clear at-home glaze, like Aveeno Living Color Shine Glaze ($6.50; drugstores), to smooth hair so it's more reflective, which instantly revs your color's vibrancy.

Giving In Gracefully

Everyone knows someone who sports a striking shade of sterling—to say nothing of Jamie Lee Curtis, Emmylou Harris, and the rest of the silver all-stars. And these gorgeous women don't lack for sex appeal (71 percent of respondents in a prevention.com poll say women with gray hair can be sexy, whereas 78 percent say the same for men). But even though many of us admire gray hair on others, we're often averse to trying out the look ourselves, according to a 2010 study in *Ageing & Society*.

Many experts wonder why. "Women can do so much to keep their faces and bodies looking young. There's no need to think gray hair will necessarily make you look older," says Rita Hazan, owner of the eponymous salon in New York City.

You can master the art of going gray gorgeously with our expert strategies and product picks for sheen, shine, and manageability.

And everyone can pull off the look, says Diana Lewis Jewell, founder of the Going Gray, Looking Great Web site (goinggraylookinggreat.com). "Women often tell me why they think gray hair won't work with their eye color or skin tone. But the fact is, for every one of those preconceived notions, there's an example to the contrary of someone who looks fabulous gray," she says. Read on for some inspiration—and a little education—if you decide to go gray.

Ease the transition. If you dye your hair, the transition to gray can be awkward. To make it smoother, ask a pro for guidance. She may suggest coloring your gray roots as they grow in with a demi-permanent dye, such as Redken Shades EQ Cover Plus (redken.com for salons), an ammonia-free color that covers up to 75 percent of gray. Once you're ready for the reveal, you just let the dye wash out. (It can take up to 28 shampoos.)

Protect your assets. Environmental pollutants and UV light can make any hair color—including barely pigmented grays—look dull. So wash about every other day (to prevent buildup) with a hydrating shampoo and conditioner containing antioxidants, which help protect against UV and environmental dam-

SHINY HAIR FROM EVERY ANGLE

Dull, drab, mousy hair ages you instantly. Here's great news: You don't need pricey products to take your hair from dull to dazzling.

Start using conditioner before and after your shampoo as a weekly treatment, says Charles Baker Strahan, hairstylist for Herbal Essences. The pre-shampoo application helps strands soak up more shine-enhancing hydrators.

Opt for foods rich in protein and omega-3 fatty acids, such as walnuts. The protein improves the health of your hair, and the fats help your scalp produce natural oils that give sheen.

Stop holding your hot tools in one spot when you're styling your hair. Heat damages the cuticle, so it doesn't lay smoothly or reflect as much light. If you use a blow-dryer or flatiron, "keep it moving at all times," says Strahan.

age. Try Giovanni Colorflage Perfectly Platinum Color Defense Shampoo and Conditioner (both $9; drugstore.com).

Get toned. Even with the right products, gray hair can take on a yellowish cast, so lather with a silver-specific shampoo once or twice a month. The classic product many stylists favor is Clairol Professional Shimmer Lights Shampoo ($9; sallybeauty.com), which has a violet toner to counteract any yellow.

Don't be blue. Use blue-hued shampoos and conditioners only once or twice a month to prevent your hair from taking on a violet cast.

Lighten up. Skip heavy pomades, waxes, and oily serums. "They can coat gray hair and make it look dusty," says Kathy Galotti, a colorist at the Rossano Ferretti Hairspa in New York City. To combat frizz, try One 'N Only Shiny Silver Ultra Shine Spray ($7; sally beauty.com), a shine spray without drying alcohol.

Polish your silver. Gray strands are usually drier than pigmented hairs, so they have a tendency to frizz and can easily look dull if you're not vigilant about upkeep. Try the tricks in this chapter for a smooth, chic look—and perennial shine.

Stay sharp. Get a modern cut with clean edges, suggests Yvette Gonzalez, senior stylist and makeup artist at Sahag Workshop in New York City. "Ask your stylist not to use a razor, because it can cause the ends to fray, making your whole style seem untidy," she says. Whatever cut you choose, be sure that you get a trim every 6 to 8 weeks. "Gray hair can start to look unruly if it's not trimmed frequently enough," says Gonzalez.

CHAPTER 29

Better Brows Now!

Don't underestimate the importance of beautiful brows. Whether yours are thinning, fading, or graying, we can help you get them in shape.

You slather on serums, touch up your grays, and sweat through hot yoga—but what have you done for your eyebrows lately? If you've never given much thought to your arches beyond the occasional tweezing, now is probably a good time to start.

"Like your skin and hair, your brows can start to show their age," says brow expert Anastasia Soare, owner of Anastasia Beverly Hills Salon. "They can thin out, become coarse and unruly, or turn gray." And just as a new haircut can trim away the years, a well-groomed, well-defined brow can lend your face a years-younger look.

ARCH ENEMY: VANISHING BROWS

The problem: "Like thinning hair, sparse brows come with age, so they make you look older than you are," says Eliza Petrescu, owner of Eliza's Eyes in New York City.

NATURAL BEAUTIES

The key to making brow pencil, powder, and gel look natural: using the right hue. "My rule of thumb is to choose a color that's a shade or two lighter than your hair," says Kristie Streicher, eyebrow expert at Warren-Tricomi Salon in Los Angeles. It ends up looking more natural, because the colors usually go on darker than you'd expect. In general, medium brown suits brunettes, warm brown is best for redheads, and taupe is best on blondes and those with gray hair. Here are three to consider.

- Lorac Creamy Brow Pencil in Brunette
- Lorac Creamy Brow Pencil in Auburn
- Lorac Creamy Brow Pencil in Blonde (each $20; sephora.com)

The solution: Use a brow powder (see "Natural Beauties" to find the right color) to fill in patchy spots and make your arches look thicker.

Your brow fix: Start by gently pulling your skin taut with one hand to create a smooth surface.

With a stiff, angled brow brush, dust on the powder in the same direction your hairs grow, using light, feathery strokes. Concentrate on sparse areas, says Kristie Streicher, eyebrow expert at Warren-Tricomi Salon in Los Angeles.

When you're finished, brush the hairs up and out with a spoolie (it's like a clean mascara wand). This blends and softens the powder so it looks more natural and removes any excess.

Must-have products: Ardell Duo Brow Brush ($4.50; sallybeauty.com) and Anastasia Brow Powder Duo ($22; sephora.com)

ARCH ENEMY: DISAPPEARING TAILS

The problem: Brows naturally thin at the outer edges (by your temples) first, but a fast fade can also be the result of overplucking. "The tail of the brow is the part that sets off the arch, which makes eyes look youthful and sexy," says

Petrescu. "Without it, eyes seem droopy and tired."

The solution: Lengthen your brow tails with pencil (see "Natural Beauties" for the right color).

Your brow fix: First, determine where the tail of your brow should end by holding a pencil diagonally from the outside corner of your nostril to the outer corner of your eye. The spot where the pencil intersects with your brow is your target.

Extend your brows to that point by using the brow pencil to sketch light, feathery strokes in the same direction your hairs grow.

Set the pencil—and blend the penciled-in tails with the rest of your hairs—by stroking a tinted brow gel over the entire length of your eyebrows.

Must-have products: CoverGirl Brow & Eye Makers Pencil ($4; drugstores) and Benefit Speed Brow Quick-Set Brow Gel ($16; benefitcosmetics.com)

AT LONG LASH

Take an eye-opening tour of these inventive mascaras—and fulfill all your fringe fantasies!

PUMP UP THE VOLUME. Deep bristles on Maybelline New York One-by-One Mascara ($8; drugstores) grab lashes for a thick, even coat.

FAN OUT. Build every lash—from corner to corner—with striking definition using L'Oreal Paris Telescopic Explosion Mascara in Carbon Black ($9.50; drugstores).

GO CURLY CUE. The bowed shape of Flirt! It Curl ($15; kohls.com) scoops up lashes, while a reservoir on the spine supplies root-to-tip coverage.

NO RUNNING! Prone to smudges under your eyes? Try stay-put CoverGirl LashBlast Volume in Waterproof ($8; drugstores).

GO LONG. Friction created by the rubberized wand of Revlon CustomEyes Mascara ($9; drugstores) gently stretches lashes to their largest. The dial adjusts to customize volume.

ARCH ENEMY: GRAYING BROWS

The problem: "From afar, gray or white brows disappear completely, which makes your features look unbalanced," Petrescu explains.

The solution: Camouflage colorless hairs using the right technique, which depends on the number of grays you have.

Your brow fix: Hide a few strays with a brow marker that matches your eyebrow color; the felt-tip point allows you to paint hairs precisely with a natural-looking color.

If you have a significant number of grays, color them temporarily by brushing on a tinted brow gel that's slightly lighter than the nongray hairs.

If your brows are mostly gray, dyeing them is the best fix. Ask your stylist if your salon offers the service (it's often free when you get your hair colored), or have it done at a spa. "Even if the hair on your head is silver or gray, I suggest dyeing brows light brown," says Petrescu. "It creates a frame for your eyes that sharpens your features for a more youthful look."

Must-have products: TouchBack BrowMarker ($20; touchbackbrow.com) and Paula Dorf Brow Tint ($20; pauladorf.com)

GROW FOR IT

If the $120 price tag of prescription lash-growth serum Latisse (or the hassle of getting a prescription) scares you off, are the more affordable, OTC lash enhancers worth a shot?

"Some nonprescription versions may stimulate growth, but they can't make this claim without being regarded as an Rx," says New York City–based dermatologist Doris Day, MD. "They can, however, provide conditioning benefits to prevent breakage and slow the fallout rate."

Try RapidLash Eyelash Enhancing Serum ($50; rapidlash.com), which claims to boost lash length 17 percent after 3 months, or Wet 'n Wild Clinical Serum ($7; Walgreens) for peptide-packed conditioning.

FABULOUS FALSIES

Glue-on lashes don't have to take you into showgirl territory. For a glamorous-yet-believable look (in less than 5 minutes), skip full lash strips and opt for shorter sections applied just to the outer corners. Bonus: The smaller size is easier to apply. We like Kre-at Beauty Half Lash Short ($15; kreatbeauty.com), which has lashes that crisscross slightly at its base—a more realistic look, as that is what lashes do naturally.

ARCH ENEMY: OVERGROWN BROWS

The problem: Bushy brows can make eyes look smaller. And longer, coarser hairs (which appear with age) might overhang at the outer edges, making lids look droopy, says Streicher.

The solution: Trim, tweeze, and set hairs in place for arches that are under control.

Your brow fix: Brush all the hairs up with a spoolie, then use brow scissors to cut the tips of hairs that extend above the top edge of the brow line, one at a time. (Cutting them all with one snip across leaves a straight edge that looks unnatural.)

Next, use slant-tip tweezers to pluck stray hairs that grow outside the swath of hair that defines your natural brow shape. "This can be tricky, so I recommend going to a pro," says Petrescu.

Finish with clear brow gel to set hairs in place without darkening them.

Must-have products: Revlon Brow Styling Gel ($6; drugstores), Tweezerman Brow Shaping Scissors & Brush ($18; tweezerman.com), and Sally Hansen Brows That Wow Diamond Slant Tip Tweezer ($13.50; drugstores)

CHAPTER 30

Undercover Agents

This generation of primers elegantly conceals flaws and delivers long-lasting, youth-boosting skin-care benefits, too.

Even if your makeup bag is very well stocked, you still might be missing one key product: a primer. Yet many makeup experts say that "not to prime is a crime."

Here's why. Whether you wear makeup regularly or not, you certainly want great skin—and that's reason enough to try one of the new high-tech primers. Worn under cosmetics (they help makeup go on smoother and last longer) or on their own, these primers create the illusion of near-perfect skin by filling in lines, hiding imperfections, and disguising pores, says Ni'Kita Wilson, a cosmetic chemist at Cosmetech Labs in Fairfield, New Jersey. Even better, the new primer formulas actually treat and heal the imperfections they hide.

"Because these primers stay on skin, using them day after day also improves your complexion over time," says Jeannette Graf, MD, a dermatologist in Great Neck, New York. No matter what your skin concern, one of these multitaskers has you covered—in a completely natural way.

YOU WANT LESS REDNESS

You need: a green-tinted primer with skin-soothing ingredients.

As we age, our skin tends to become redder, according to Dr. Graf, who blames cumulative sun exposure and sensitivity. The fix? A primer with a green tint, which counteracts redness so it's less noticeable. Try Fusion Beauty Prime Results Anti-Redness Primer ($42; fusionbeauty.com), which has a mineral-rich algae that protects skin from stressors that cause redness and irritation.

If your redness is due to rosacea, choose a primer that also has sunscreen, since sun exposure can exacerbate the condition. Try Clinique Redness Solutions Daily Protective Base SPF 15 ($18.50; clinique.com).

How to: Use a sponge to apply a dab over any red areas and blend well. You can follow up with foundation or concealer, but even without makeup, you'll see an improvement.

YOU WANT A MORE EVEN-TONED COMPLEXION

You need: a primer that targets discoloration.

If you have dark spots, look for a primer with niacinamide, which is a vitamin that helps lighten pigmented areas by preventing melanin from traveling

PUT THE BRAKES ON BROWN SPOTS

A surprising cause of spots has surfaced: Women exposed to higher concentrations of traffic-related particles had 20 percent more age spots. A study in the *Journal of Investigative Dermatology* suggests these particles may ramp up melanin production.

If you live near traffic—or spend a lot of time in it—use lotion with ingredients that inhibit melanin, such as licorice root extract, kojic acid, and niacinamide. Try PCA Skin Perfecting Protection SPF 30 ($24; 877-722-7546 for locations) or Neutrogena Tone Correcting Daily Moisture SPF 30 from Ageless Intensives ($19; drugstores).

into skin cells, according to Carolyn Jacob, MD, director of Chicago Cosmetic Surgery and Dermatology. An especially good one is CoverGirl & Olay Simply Ageless Serum Primer ($14; drugstores).

If your skin is dull all over, go for a primer with light-reflecting particles, such as L'Oreal Paris Studio Secrets Professional Anti-Dull Skin Primer ($13; drugstores), a sheer peachy-pink tint that can be worn alone (it works best on light to medium skin tones) or as an illuminating base for foundation.

How to: Use fingers to blend a thin layer all over your face, suggests Los Angeles–based makeup artist Toby Fleischman.

YOU WANT CLEARER SKIN

You need: a primer that controls oil and acne.

Products like Philosophy On A Clear Day Acne Clarifying Primer ($30; philosophy.com) and BareMinerals Prime Time Oil Control Foundation Primer ($22; sephora.com) contain blemish-healing ingredients like salicylic acid. They also create a soft, matte finish so skin looks prettier while the acne fixers do their job.

If you want to follow with foundation, these formulas also prevent the makeup slippage that is common with oily skin.

How to: Use a sponge to apply them because, says Fleischman, "oil and bacteria on fingers can make problem skin worse."

YOU WANT FEWER FINE LINES

You need: a line-plumping primer with built-in anti-agers.

This class of primers has moisturizing ingredients to temporarily fill in fine lines, so they're less noticeable. As for skin care benefits, some, like Sonia Kashuk Primer Vitamin Serum ($18; Target), contain antioxidants to protect skin against the aging effects of free radicals. Others, such as Peter Thomas Roth Un-Wrinkle Primer ($38; peterthomasroth.com), have peptides to stimulate collagen production.

How to: Smooth a pea-size dollop all over your face, as if you were applying moisturizer, and follow with makeup.

YOU WANT BRIGHTER-LOOKING EYES

You need: eyelid primer.

You don't have to wear eye shadow to reap the benefits of these primers. The formulas go on creamy but dry to a matte finish that balances out the color of your eyelids and helps eye makeup stay on longer without creasing. Both Glo Minerals Lid Primer ($24; gloskincare.com) and Laura Geller Waterproof Eye Spackle ($22; qvc.com) have a slight golden-beige tint (it won't affect the color of your eye shadow) to neutralize the blue and pink tones on lids that can make you look tired.

How to: Use your ring or middle finger to blend a small amount of primer all over clean, dry lids.

BONUS! DOUBLE-DUTY BEAUTY FOODS

The following nutritious foods are a recipe for great hair, glowing skin, and more—whether you eat them or turn them into topical treatments.

One quick caveat: Before using foods or beverages on skin or hair, do a patch test. Prepare the item as suggested, swab a bit on the inside of your wrist, then wait 48 hours to see if you develop a reaction. If not, proceed.

Avocado

Eat it. Consider avocado the overachiever of beauty superfoods. It's rich in protective antioxidants and essential fatty acids, which help keep skin plump and smooth, says New York City dietitian Shari Bilt Boockvar, RD. Eating the fruit can also help replenish the protective layer of fatty acids that surrounds skin cells, keeping moisture in and preventing dehydration, according to Jessica Wu, MD, assistant clinical professor of dermatology at the University of Southern California Medical School in Los Angeles and author of *Feed Your Face*. Get your avocado fix by using it in place of mayo on a sandwich, or whip half an avocado and add it to your smoothie or salad dressing recipes.

Apply it. "An avocado face mask may help slow skin's aging process," says nutritionist Lisa Drayer, RD, who points to a 2006 study published in *Phytotherapy Research* that found that applying avocado oil to skin can stimulate col-

WAKE-UP MAKEUP

Whether you had a restless night or always seem to look like it, you can perk up your entire eye area in a wink. Blend a champagne highlighter from just under your brows out to and over your temples, suggests Physicians Formula makeup artist Joanna Schlip.

"The highlighter reflects light on an area usually sunken in shadow, giving eyes an instant lift," she explains. Try Shiseido Makeup Accentuating Color Stick in Champagne Flush ($33; shiseido.com), or Physicians Formula Powder Palette Mineral Glow Pearls with brush ($14; drugstores).

lagen and elastin production. Make an anti-aging moisturizing mask by pureeing a ripe avocado and mixing it with ¼ cup sour cream, which has lactic acid to help exfoliate dead skin cells. Spread over your face and leave on for 10 minutes before rinsing with water.

Tea

Drink it. All teas boast skin-boosting antioxidants, but green and white varieties are especially good because they have double the antioxidants of black tea as well as EGCG (epigallocatechin gallate), which is a type of antioxidant that "protects skin from damage caused by exposure to sun and pollutants," says Dr. Wu. Sip up—but cook with the brew too. It makes a great poaching liquid for chicken or fish.

Apply it. Tea is a natural hair-color booster that can function as a rinse to bring out highlights in dyed or undyed hair, says Jet Rhys, owner of the Jet Rhys Salons in San Diego. Chamomile revitalizes golden highlights in blonde hair, black tea perks up brunettes, and berry or red teas add oomph to auburn or red hair. Prepare 8 ounces, let it cool, and then saturate your strands with the solution. Put on a shower cap and wait for 15 to 30 minutes, and then rinse with water.

IN THE CLEAR

Picture someone with acne—go ahead, we'll wait. Got an image in mind? Chances are you conjured visions of the teen next door or that pimply boy from high school. But experts say the face of acne is changing, and these days, it looks more like . . . you. Research shows 35 percent of women in their thirties, 26 percent in their forties, and 15 percent age 50+ battle breakouts.

Adult-Acne Instigators

Here are four common triggers of grown-up pimple problems.

HORMONAL CHANGES: Whenever your body experiences a spike in "male" hormones such as testosterone, oil production increases—and that can cause a clogged pore where *P. acnes* bacteria grows, leading to inflammation and pimples. This may occur more frequently during perimenopause, but it also happens just before your period. (Women over the age of 33 are more likely to get premenstrual pimples than younger women are, according to one study.)

YOUR DIET: Greasy food doesn't cause a greasy face, but the following foods might exacerbate an already-brewing condition.

- **SIMPLE CARBS AND SUGAR:** Any food that leads to a spike in your blood sugar (such as pasta, bread, and sweets) can trigger skin's inflammatory response and provoke a breakout, according to Linda K. Franks, MD, a dermatologist in New York City.
- **DAIRY:** Several studies have shown a link between dairy products and pimples, perhaps because of the hormones that are present in these foods. Buying organic can help: Traditional dairy products can come from hormone-fed animals, so they often have more hormones than their organic counterparts.
- **CHOCOLATE:** A small study presented at the February 2011 meeting of the Academy of Dermatology found a correlation between the amount of chocolate that participants consumed (only men were studied, so as to minimize the role of hormonal influence) and the number of acne lesions they developed.

STRESS: If the thought of cutting back on chocolate stresses you out, though, please relax! Experts say stress can lead to acne by signaling the release of cortisol, a hormone that tells your body to produce more pore-clogging oil.

MEDICAL CONDITIONS: Health issues with a hormonal component, such as high testosterone levels or polycystic ovarian syndrome, are often-overlooked causes of acne.

"PCOS affects 5 to 10 percent of women, and many of them suffer for years without realizing they have it," says Mitch Chasin, MD, the medical director of Reflections Center for Skin & Body in Livingston, New Jersey. If your acne is accompanied by excessive hair growth or irregular periods, it's worth talking to your doctor, who may do a blood test or ultrasound to determine whether or not you have PCOS. If you do, the condition—and other types of hormone imbalances—can often be treated with a medication such as an oral contraceptive or antiandrogen.

Adult-Only Acne Zappers

Some pimple products contain benzoyl peroxide, which can dry mature skin. Instead, try these treatments. Head to the dermatologist if you don't see improvement in 4 weeks.

BORBA PMS SKIN RESCUE 7-DAY TREATMENT SYSTEM ($26; drugstores) fights hormonal blemishes with individually packaged day and night treatment ampoules.

MURAD ACNE & WRINKLE REDUCER ($58; sephora.com) has salicylic acid to help clear pimples, along with anti-aging retinol that works on fine lines.

NELSONS PURE & CLEAR PURIFYING CLEANSING WIPES ($8; Whole Foods) freshen skin with a pimple-fighting witch hazel–based solution.

CLEARASIL ULTRA RAPID ACTION SEAL-TO-CLEAR GEL ($10; drugstores) heals with salicylic acid and forms an invisible protective film over pimples. (It's great under makeup!)

Almonds

Eat them. Going gray? Reach for these nuts. According to Dr. Wu, almonds contain high levels of catalase, which is an enzyme that might help slow the graying process by preventing a buildup of hydrogen peroxide in follicles that can cause hair to turn gray. Almonds aren't just a snack, though: Pulverize them in a food processor and add to waffle batter, or use as a crunchy coating for chicken.

Apply them. Go nuts for this exfoliating body scrub recipe from Kym Douglas, the author of *The Beauty Cookbook*: Grind ¼ cup almonds in a food processor until superfine, then mix in 2 tablespoons organic virgin coconut oil to make a paste. In the shower, rub the skin-softening mixture over rough areas, such as knees and elbows, and then rinse with water.

Cocoa

Eat it. "Cocoa has a high concentration of flavanols, plant compounds with antioxidant properties that help protect skin from sun damage," says Dr. Wu. Add a tablespoon of 70 percent cocoa powder to a cup of barbecue sauce for richer flavor.

Apply it. Here's a no-cal way to get the skin benefits of cocoa's flavanols. Use it as a bath soak, suggests Ginger McLean, former spa director for the Spa at the Hotel Hershey in Pennsylvania. To do, add ⅛ cup unsweetened cocoa powder, which also nourishes dry skin, and ⅓ cup instant fat-free dry milk to your tub.

A BRIGHT IDEA TO HIDE DARK CIRCLES

It doesn't get simpler than this: Let under-eye concealer sit on your skin for a full minute before blending it in.

"This allows some moisture to evaporate from the formula, so it's more opaque and covers better," says makeup artist Renee Ryan of Cargo Cosmetics in Toronto. Look for one with antioxidants or peptides that hides and treats circles. Here's one to try: NYC New York Color Smooth Skin Liquid Concealer ($4; drugstores).

Yogurt

Eat it. Get ready to show off your pearly whites! Spooning up yogurt can help keep your grin gorgeous. "It has calcium and phosphorus that can strengthen tooth enamel and protect your teeth from cavities," says Drayer. What's more, varieties such as Greek yogurt are high in protein, which is an essential nutrient for the production of collagen, a fibrous substance that keeps your skin youthful looking, according to Dr. Wu. Score more daily dairy by replacing regular sour cream with fat-free plain yogurt in recipes for salad dressings.

Apply it. Yogurt contains lactic acid, an alpha hydroxy that's great for sloughing away dead skin cells and unclogging pores, says Dr. Wu. She suggests using full-fat plain yogurt as a mask: Apply a thin layer to clean skin and leave on for 10 minutes before rinsing. You can also whip it into a protein-rich hair mask, says Rhys. Whisk together ½ cup full-fat yogurt, 3 tablespoons honey, and 1 egg yolk. Apply to hair, put on a shower cap, and wait 15 minutes before rinsing and washing as usual.

Strawberries

Eat them. "Strawberries pack the double punch of high levels of vitamin C and ellagic acid," says Howard Murad, MD, FAAD, associate clinical professor of dermatology at UCLA's Geffen School of Medicine. Vitamin C is essential for the production of collagen and acts as an antioxidant to prevent environmental damage. And a 2007 study in the *American Journal of Clinical Nutrition* showed that high intake of vitamin C was associated with a lower likelihood of wrinkles and skin dryness.

Apply them. Studies show that both ellagic acid and vitamin C in strawberries help protect skin from environmental damage, so using strawberries as part of an at-home beauty treatment could be beneficial. Try this face mask recipe from Douglas: Puree the berries in a blender and mix in chilled full-fat plain yogurt and a squirt of lemon juice. (It has antiseptic properties and may help lighten dark spots.) Apply the mixture to your face, leave it on for 20 minutes, then rinse.

Ellagic acid increases skin's ability to hold moisture and, says Dr. Wu, has been shown to help fade dark spots caused by sun exposure. A new way to work the fruit into your menu: Add a touch of balsamic vinegar to pureed strawberries and use the mixture as a sweet sauce for grilled chicken.

Coffee

Sip it. Coffee is a well-known pick-me-up, but a cup of joe can perk up skin too. "It has antioxidants to help protect skin from sun damage and help prevent the breakdown of collagen and elastin that leads to wrinkles and sagging," according to Dr. Murad. Aim for no more than one 8-ounce cup a day, because coffee in large doses can dehydrate skin. Another way to enjoy more of the buzzy beans: Use finely ground coffee as part of a spice rub for steak or beef.

Apply it. The caffeine that's in coffee is a topical diuretic (it pulls water out of skin), so it can help depuff eyelids and is often used as an ingredient in cellulite creams because it temporarily gives skin a smoother appearance, says Dr. Murad. Douglas recommends using cooled coffee grounds as a scrub on thighs and buttocks, where cellulite tends to appear.

"The scrubbing stimulates circulation, and the caffeine in the grounds has a temporary shrinking effect on the cellulite," she explains. A coffee rinse can also deepen and richen the hue of brown hair, says Rhys. Brew 2 cups of strong coffee and allow it to cool. In the shower, shampoo, squeeze out excess moisture, pour the cooled coffee over strands, and put on a shower cap. At the end of your shower, rinse, then condition as usual.

Water

Sip it. If you're hydrated (and you are if your urine is pale yellow every time you pee), there's no proof that gulping more water does anything for your skin. But "if your skin cells aren't able to retain moisture well, your complexion can still become dehydrated," says dermatologist Howard Murad, MD, author of *The Water Secret.*

How do you get cells to hang on to water? Load up on raw fruits and vegetables. Thanks to an added boost of important antioxidants, fiber, and other nutrients, they help your body retain H_2O longer than if you simply drank water.

Apply it. Try these hydrating, spa-inspired treatments for gorgeous skin.

Soften up, head to toe. Wet your skin in the shower, then turn off the spray and combine equal parts organic, unprocessed sea salt and a shower gel that doubles as a moisturizing lotion: Try Olay Purely Pristine Moisturizing Body Wash ($4; drugstores). Massage the mixture all over, concentrating on rough spots—the salt acts as a manual exfoliant, removing dead skin so the moisturizers can better penetrate. Rinse to reveal soft, hydrated skin.

Clear your complexion (and your sinuses!) Turn your bathroom into a steam room by placing a Level Naturals Shower Bomb ($8 for four; levelnaturals.com) on the floor of your tub before you shower. As the warm water hits it, the tablet melts, releasing steam laden with blemish-fighting tea tree oil, plus sinus-clearing eucalyptus and menthol vapor.

Heal dry, itchy skin. Draw a warm bath, adding a can (13.5 ounces) of organic, unsweetened coconut milk to the running water. "It's loaded with beneficial fats that hydrate skin," says Kristin Carpenter, spa director at Eau Spa at the Ritz-Carlton in Palm Beach, FL. Soak for 10 to 15 minutes, then pat dry. While skin is still slightly damp, apply a vitamin-rich body lotion such as Jergens Ultra Healing Extra Dry Skin Moisturizer ($5; drugstores) with vitamins C, E, and B_5.

Set the right temperature. One water temperature does not suit all beauty rituals. Here, experts explain when it's best to turn up (or down) the heat.

Ice cold: Speed up polish drying time with a 1-minute soak in icy water, suggests Kristin Carpenter, spa director at Eau Spa at the Ritz-Carlton in Palm Beach, Florida.

Cold: Remove cleanser with cold water to temporarily make pores look smaller. The temp also constricts blood vessels slightly to reduce redness, says Meryl Joerg, MD, a dermatologist at Advanced Dermatology PC in New York City.

Tepid: Rinse out hair conditioner with lukewarm water. "It closes the cuticle so strands look shinier and are less prone to frizz," explains Carpenter.

Warm: Shower in just-warm-enough water. "Prolonged exposure to hot water weakens skin's protective barrier that locks in moisture," says Amy Wechsler, MD, a dermatologist in New York City.

Hot: Wet skin with hot water before shaving to soften hair fibers and plump follicles so hairs stand up straighter. "You'll get a much closer shave," promises Carpenter.

CHAPTER 31

No More Excuses

Sixty-nine percent of women lie to themselves, saying that they don't need sunscreen. Don't be one of them. Arm yourself with the simplest and strongest weapon that we have against wrinkles, age spots, and skin cancer.

Despite the fact that most women know they should wear sunscreen every day of the year, only 31 percent do, according to a recent poll by Prevention.com. And many of those who skip SPF feel guilty about it—so much so that 31 percent admit they've fibbed about putting on sunscreen because they're embarrassed about their bad habit.

So what gives? If we all know that sunscreen helps to protect our skin from cancer and prevent signs of aging such as spots and wrinkles, why aren't more of us using it?

To find out, *Prevention* asked dermatologists to share some of the most common excuses women give for going outdoors unprotected. Read on and you'll discover there's really no good reason to skimp on sunscreen. You'll be healthier (and younger looking!) if you use it.

EXCUSE #1

"The chemicals in sunscreen are probably more dangerous than sun exposure."

Reality check: Sunscreens have gotten some bad press lately, including claims that they contain cancer-causing ingredients. But a recently published review of the studies on which these claims are based should ease fears.

"Many of the safety concerns are not well founded. They're based on petri dish or animal data that doesn't relate to humans," says Steven Wang, MD, director of dermatologic surgery at Memorial Sloan-Kettering Cancer Center in Basking Ridge, New Jersey, and coauthor of the review. For example, in one study, mice fed a whopping dose of oxybenzone, a UV-light absorber commonly found in sunscreens, exhibited estrogenic effects, which the researchers believe could cause cancer cells to grow more rapidly. But by Dr. Wang's calculations, it would take more than 250 years for someone who uses sunscreen daily to be exposed to the amount of oxybenzone used in the study.

Still worried? Use a sunscreen such as Beyond Coastal Natural Sunscreen SPF 30+ ($16; beyondcoastal.com), which has zinc oxide and titanium dioxide in lieu of chemical sunscreens.

BURN NOTICE

Despite your best efforts, you might still burn. Here's how to heal.

Pop an aspirin immediately to help with the pain and decrease inflammation so your skin won't get as red.

Drink 8 glasses of water a day over the next 48 hours. Water cools you from the inside out and helps stave off dehydration (you lose moisture through burned skin).

Soothe skin and speed healing by soaking a cloth in anti-inflammatory witch hazel and applying it to the affected area. Dickinson's Original Witch Hazel Oil Controlling Towelettes ($5; drugstores) work well for this purpose too.

EXCUSE #2

"I don't get a lot of sun."

Reality check: You don't have to be on the beach to soak up rays. Most people rack up 14 hours of casual UV exposure per week. And in one study, short spurts of UVA light twice a week resulted in significant damage to the fibers that keep skin smooth and firm in just 12 weeks. Makeup and a daily lotion with SPF are great steps, but "the protection is short-lived on hot, sunny days," says New York City dermatologist Arielle Kauvar, MD. Use a sweat-resistant sunscreen with at least SPF 30 on all sun-exposed areas to be safe.

EXCUSE #3

"It's a drag to reapply sunscreen."

Reality check: Five minutes every 2 hours—that's all it takes to apply the 1 ounce (2 tablespoons) of sunscreen recommended for protection when you're in a bathing suit or outdoors for extended periods. And when it's time to reapply, new sprays like Aveeno Hydrosport Sunblock Spray SPF 85 ($10; drugstores) make it less of a hassle and even adhere to wet skin. Easy, right?

EXCUSE #4

"Sunscreen is too expensive."

Reality check: As long as you pick one that clearly states it blocks both UVA and UVB rays, there's no need to break the bank when buying.

"Research doesn't show any relationship between price and protection," reports Dr. Wang. Try Banana Boat Ultra Defense SPF 30 Continuous Clear Spray ($10; drugstores).

EXCUSE #5

"I don't need sunscreen because my skin is naturally dark."

Reality check: "Skin cancer is color-blind," warns Jeanine Downie, MD, a dermatologist in Montclair, New Jersey, and coauthor of *Beautiful Skin of Color*. In fact, skin cancer rates are increasing among Latinos—many of whom have dark skin. Mixed racial heritage may be one reason for the rise, says Vivian Bucay, MD, clinical assistant professor at the University of Texas Health Science Center in San Antonio.

"Hispanics are more genetically diverse than other groups, so even if they have dark skin, they could burn just as someone with fair German or Irish skin would," she says. Plus, those with dark skin may not recognize skin cancers as early in their development as people with light skin. (One study found advanced stages of melanoma at time of diagnosis in 18 percent of Hispanics and 26 percent of African Americans, compared with 12 percent of Caucasians.)

If that's not reason enough for SPF, Dr. Downie has one more: Sun deepens dark spots common in all women of color. Her protection pick: sheer, nonchalky Neutrogena Ultra Sheer Dry-Touch Sunblock SPF 30 ($10; neutrogena.com).

EXCUSE #6

"I look so good with a tan."

Reality check: Think long-term: Saggy, leathery skin is not pretty. Instead, try the subtle sheen of Hawaiian Tropic Shimmer Effect Lotion Sunscreen SPF 40 ($9; drugstores).

EXCUSE #7

"I haven't gotten burned yet."

Reality check: "This is the skin equivalent of 'I've never had a car wreck, so I don't need a seat belt,'" says Ranella Hirsch, MD, a dermatologist in Boston. Though a cavalier attitude toward sunscreen might not be a big deal when you're young, skin loses its ability to produce melanin effectively as you get older, and that might actually make you more likely to burn. The fact is, sun damage—including wrinkles and loss of firmness—occurs whether or not you're seeing red. And that's a good reason to use a sunscreen like Avon Anew Solar Advance Sunscreen Body Lotion SPF 30 ($24; avon.com); it prevents burning and helps to heal past damage with a blend of antioxidant-rich botanicals.

GET GLOWING

A diet packed with carotenoid-rich produce (such as tomatoes, carrots, and peaches) actually gives your skin a golden hue that makes you more attractive, according to a study in the journal *Evolution and Human Behavior*. Scientists believe that this subtle signal of robust good health helped our ancestors find the fittest mates, and the preference still draws us to someone with a luminous skin tone. So skip the tanning bed and head to the farmers' market for a healthy, sun-free way to glow.

EXCUSE #8

"Skin cancer is one of the most treatable forms of cancer."

Reality check: UVB rays lead to the development of the two most common types of skin cancer, basal cell carcinoma and squamous cell carcinoma, and UVA rays penetrate deeper into the skin, triggering melanoma, the deadliest form of skin cancer. While it's true that melanoma is usually curable when caught early, it still kills 8,000 Americans a year. And those who are lucky enough to recover from skin cancer aren't necessarily unscathed.

Take basal cell carcinomas, for instance: "They penetrate deeply, and slowly destroy healthy tissue," explains Andrew Kaufman, MD, clinical associate professor of dermatology at the David Geffen School of Medicine at UCLA. Both the biopsy and the surgery to remove the lesions can leave a scar or, in rare cases, disfigurement.

Still not screaming for sunscreen? A number of studies also show that having skin cancer increases your risk of developing other cancers, including breast, non-Hodgkin's lymphoma, lung, and kidney. Here's one explanation: "Even a little UV light can weaken cells in the skin and compromise your immune surveillance," says Dr. Bucay. "It's like removing the security guards from a bank and allowing the robbers to come in."

CHAPTER 32

The Pedi-Cure

No matter the weather, or season, anytime is time to treat yourself to an all-natural, at-home pedicure.

Polished toes look great peeping out of sandals, but a pedicure can do more than just pretty up your feet. If you incorporate massage, you'll also get health benefits such as improved circulation, anxiety reduction, and pain relief, according to several studies. And the good news is, you don't have to go to a nail salon and expose your feet to sketchy-looking footbaths and communal tools to get these benefits. Use this expert-approved plan and do it in the comfort of your own home.

STEP 1: CLIP AND FILE

Start by taking off old polish with a nonacetone remover. You've probably heard that acetone dries out your nails, but breathing in the fumes can also cause throat irritation and even increase your pulse rate, according to the National Institutes of Health. Instead, try Karma Organic Nail Polish Remover with Soybean Oil & Lavender ($12; karmaorganicspa.com).

Next, use a pair of nail clippers to trim your nails straight across, then file the edges smooth.

"It's tempting to trim and file toenails into the same squoval that's popular for fingernails, but the rounded shape can lead to ingrown toenails," says Kim D'Amato, founder of New York City's Priti Organic Spa.

"I also recommend using a glass nail file, which is easy to disinfect."

Try the Swissco Emery Glass Nail File ($7.50; sallybeauty.com).

STEP 2: SUBMERGE AND SOOTHE

A foot soak is more than an excuse to relax.

"It softens calluses, so they're easier to remove," says manicurist Nausil Zaheer, owner of Karma Organic Spa, a natural nail salon in New Jersey.

Here's how to do it: Dip your feet in a basin of warm water for 3 minutes; add 1 ounce of a foot soak such as Ahava Lavender Mineral Bath Salts ($22; ahavaus.com) for extra skin-softening power. Next, rub a pumice, like the Tweezerman Pedro Callus Stone ($20; tweezerman.com), over rough spots. Skip the callus shavers or razors, advises Zaheer: "Doing your own feet, it's hard to hold them at the right angle, and you can easily take off too much skin or cut yourself."

NAIL SALON 911

Don't want to do your own nails? When you visit a salon, take health matters into your own hands (and feet!) by following these tips to ensure your salon is safe.

GIVE IT THE ONCE-OVER. If there's no time to sweep the floor, nail dryers may be dirty too. Up-to-date licenses for all the technicians should be visibly posted.

ASK HOW TOOLS ARE DISINFECTED. FDA–approved steam pressurized sterilizers (or autoclaves) are best. Soaking tools may not be as effective if the disinfecting solution isn't fresh.

SCAN BEFORE YOU SOAK. Make sure the footbaths are drained and cleaned between each client, because they can contain harmful bacteria.

HELPING HANDS

Is your skin drier than the Sahara? When hands are bone-dry, "your goal is to both restore moisture and rebuild skin's protective barrier layer," says New York City–based dermatologist Diane Berson, MD. Here's how:

STEP 1: EXFOLIATE. Slough with a gentle scrub such as Freeman Bare Hands Hand & Cuticle Renewal Scrub ($4; drugstores) to help moisturizers penetrate.

STEP 2: SLATHER. Aveda Hand Relief ($7.50; aveda.com) has glycerin and plant oils to quench skin, plus fatty acids to condition the skin's barrier.

STEP 3: WRAP. Cotton gloves (or even plastic wrap) lock in moisture while body heat speeds treatment.

STEP 3: MOISTURIZE AND MASSAGE

Rinse your feet, then rub in a dollop of moisturizing foot cream, such as Collective Wellbeing Foot Butter ($11.50; collectivewellbeing.com).

Even an amateur masseuse can reduce stress levels in as little as 5 minutes: Knead along the center of your foot, concentrating on tense muscles.

STEP 4: PREP AND POLISH

Use a cuticle pusher to gently push back cuticles.

"It's safer than trimming with a nipper, which can nick skin and invite infection," Zaheer says.

Next, apply one layer of a base coat, such as Dermelect Cosmeceuticals Makeover Ridge Filler ($18; dermelect.com). The formula uses peptides to make nails stronger and healthier. Let it dry for a minute, and then brush on two layers of polish. D'Amato suggests products without dibutyl phthalate (DBP), toluene, or formaldehyde—which are potentially harmful in large doses, says the Environmental Working Group. Finish with a UV-protecting topcoat, like Orly Sunscreen for Nails ($10; orlybeauty.com).

CHAPTER 33

Scentsational Scents

Perfume is nothing to sniff at: A new fragrance can improve your mood, slim you down, and update your image. Put some spring in your scent!

Have you been wearing the same scent since shoulder pads were in style—the first time around? Your nose may have adapted to it.

"When your brain smells an aroma frequently enough, it no longer perceives it as worth paying attention to," explains Stephen Warrenburg, PhD, a research fellow at International Flavors and Fragrances in Union Beach, New Jersey.

That's reason enough to update your signature scent, but many fragrance makers are giving you another: new scents that play down heavier notes but smell similar to classics you love. Frequently nuanced with airy florals such as lily of the valley, freesia, and honeysuckle or notes like clementine, orange, mandarin, and grapefruit, these new blends "deliver a burst of freshness when you spray them on," says Natasha Cote, a perfumer at Givaudan in New York City. Consider the following scents for what ails you.

CAN PERFUME PEEL OFF POUNDS?

In a study done by Alan Hirsch, MD, neurological director of the Smell and Taste Treatment and Research Foundation in Chicago, people who smelled green apple, banana, or peppermint several times daily lost an average of 30 pounds in 6 months.

"We think the scents may curb cravings," Dr. Hirsch says. Harvey Prince Eau De Lite ($55; harveyprince.com), which features all three notes, could do the same.

IF YOU NEED A MOOD MAKEOVER

Sniffing something pleasant is a faster way to cheer up than, say, looking at a treasured souvenir or hearing a favorite song.

"The olfactory system is like an interstate highway connection to the emotional part of the brain, while our visual and auditory systems are more like country roads," says Charles Wysocki, PhD, a behavioral neuroscientist at Monell Chemical Senses Center in Philadelphia.

Research shows the cheeriest scents might be citrus. In fact, one study at Ohio State University found that sniffing lemon oil can improve your mood and boost the release of norepinephrine, a mood-regulating hormone.

Here are two scents to make you smile: C.O. Bigelow Lemon Eau de Parfum ($34.50 for 3.4 ounces; cobigelow.com) and Origins Gloomaway Grapefruit Body Mist ($28; origins.com).

IF YOU WANT A UNIQUE
SCENT MADE JUST FOR YOU

One scent does not fit all, which is why you might consider custom blending your own. At Aveda stores, choose from 12 essential oil blends to create a Personal Blend Aroma, and then infuse your DIY formula into a spray-on fragrance, moisturizer, or body wash (prices start at $11; find a store near you at aveda.com).

For a fun way to mix it up at home, check out Melange Perfumes Solid Perfume Blending Palettes ($28; melangeperfume.com). Each CD–size case contains four solid perfumes that you can layer on your skin for a completely personalized blend.

IF YOU'RE NOT A "PERFUME PERSON"

If you've never found a fragrance you like, try one that smells like you—only better. As Boulder, Colorado, perfumer Dawn Hurwitz explains (and all dog owners know!), every person emits a distinct scent affected by genetics and

A NOSE FOR NATURALS

When you're interested in natural beauty alternatives, choosing a new perfume can be tricky. Most scents, even the ones boasting natural-sounding notes such as lavender or herbs, are a complex mix of synthetic chemicals combined in a lab to mimic smells found in nature. And because fragrance formulas are proprietary, companies aren't required to disclose their formulas, making it hard to know what's truly natural.

But now perfumers are producing delicious, complex scents using only flower extracts and plant alcohols, and many print their entire ingredient list on the label to prove it. Check out the following options.

GIORGIO ARMANI ACQUA DI GIOIA ($62 for 1.7 ounces; giorgioarmanibeauty. com) has a jasmine note similar to the one in Acqua di Gio's classic blend, plus a kick of crushed mint and Italian lemon zest.

LANCOME TRESOR IN LOVE ($55 for 1.7 ounces; department stores) features the rosy notes of the original Tresor, combined with fruity nectarine, bergamot, and pear.

YVES SAINT LAURENT BELLE D'OPIUM ($69 for 1.6 ounces; yslbeautyus.com), with peach, Casablanca lily, and gardenia, is lighter but just as delectable as the original amber-based Opium scent.

diet, among other things. While some notes, such as rose, stand up to our natural scents, others, including certain musks, smell different on almost everyone.

Armed with this knowledge, Hurwitz, who creates custom perfumes, developed a tester blend with a musklike note that she sprays on clients' skin to judge how their scent will affect a perfume. When she realized that many women liked the tester almost as much as their custom scent, she bottled it as Dawn Spencer Hurwitz Special Formula X ($80 for 1 ounce; dshperfumes.com), which smells different on everyone and isn't remotely perfume-y.

Parisian fragrance company Juliette Has A Gun has developed a scent that works similarly and tellingly christened it Not A Perfume ($85 for 1.7 ounces; luckyscent.com). Its single note, Ambroxan, gives off a unique, subtly musky aroma. Bonus: "Warm skin intensifies Ambroxan's aroma, so it lingers," says Stephen Nilsen, a perfumer at Givaudan.

PRETTY, HEALTHY PERFUME

If you have dry skin, perfumes can be irritating because they often contain ethanol, which disturbs naturally occurring fatty acids that help skin cells retain moisture. To smell heavenly and keep skin healthy, try ethanol-free scents like Lush Gorilla Solid Perfumes ($10 to $16 each; lushusa.com) or Lisa Hoffman Beauty Fragrance Bracelets ($60 each; hsn.com), which have refillable charms to hold scented pellets that never touch your skin.

HOW TO SMELL YOUNGER

Beauty may be in the eye of the beholder, but according to a study by the Smell and Taste Treatment and Research Foundation in Chicago, age might be in the nose. Women wearing a grapefruity fragrance were perceived by men as being an average of 6 years younger.

"Citrus scents boost your mood," says neurological director Alan Hirsch, MD. So feeling happy may make men look at some women as being younger. Try Clarins Eau des Jardins ($50; clarins.com) or Dove Go Fresh Energizing Body Mist ($4; drugstores).

PHOTO CREDITS

Pages 89-102: ©Terry Doyle

Pages 183-188: ©Rus Anson

Pages 195-197: ©Chris Philpot

Pages 203-209: ©Christa Renee

Pages 213-217: ©Michael Darter

INDEX

Underscored page references indicate boxed text and tables.
Boldface references indicate photographs and illustrations.

Appearance, discomfort with, 307

Apples, 160
　Apple-Cherry Pie, 160
　Apple Sausage Penne, 150
　"Baked" Apple Halves with Maple
　　Cream, 165
　Baked German Apple Pancake with
　　Cherry Preserves, 124
　Waldorf Apple Salad, 132

Apricots
　Couscous with Chickpeas, Dried Fruit,
　　and Cilantro, 152
　Fancy Fruit Tart, 157

Arches, effect of shoes on, 174, 175, 176, 179

Ardell Duo Brow Brush, 320

Aromatase inhibitors (AIs), joint pain
　　from, 57–58

Arthritis. *See* Osteoarthritis

Artichokes
　Mediterranean Pizza, 154
　Stuffed Artichokes, 139

Asics Gel-Tech Walker Neo 2 athletic
　　shoe, 178

Asparagus, 135
　Asparagus-Avocado Soup, 135

Aspirin, 13, 24, 338

Athletic first-position biceps curl, in Ballet
　　Boot Camp Challenge, 184, **184**

Athletic shoes
　recommended brands of, 178–79
　when to replace, 177

Atrial fibrillation, yoga for, 54–55

Aveda Hand Relief, 345

Aveda Personal Blend Aroma, 348

Aveeno Hydrosport Sunblock Spray SPF
　　85, 339

Aveeno Living Color Shine Glaze, 315

Avocado
　Asparagus-Avocado Soup, 135
　as beauty food, 328–29

Avon Anew Clinical Luminosity Pro
　　Brightening Hand Cream SPF 15,
　　304

Avon Anew Solar Advance Sunscreen
　　Body Lotion SPF 30, 340

B

Back fat, reducing, 203–4, **203–4**, 208

Back pain treatments, 56, 58, 61

Ballet Boot Camp Challenge
　components of, 181
　exercises in, 183–88, **183–88**
　guidelines and gear for, 183
　results from, 181–82, 185, 188
　schedule for, 182, 182
　video of, 188

Ballet leg lift, in Ballet Boot Camp
　　Challenge, 186, **186**

Bamboo bedding, 287

Banana Boat Ultra Defense SPF 30
　　Continuous Clear Spray, 339

Bananas
　Fruit Freeze, 166

Bandages, for blisters, 24

Barbecue sauce
　BBQ Chicken Sliders, 236

BareMinerals Prime Time Oil Control
　　Foundation Primer, 327

Basal cell carcinoma, 341

Basil
　Beans with Herbed Tomatoes and Goat
　　Cheese, 141

Bathing, dry skin from, 301

Bath soak, cocoa, 332

Beans
　Beans with Herbed Tomatoes and Goat
　　Cheese, 141
　Black Bean Burgers, 77
　bloating from, 219
　White Bean "BLT" Tartine, 156

Frozen treats, recommended, 250–51
Fruits. *See also specific fruits*
    as Active Calorie food, 68, 69
    bloating from, 219
    Breakfast Parfaits, 123
    Couscous with Chickpeas, Dried Fruit,
        and Cilantro, 152
    Fancy Fruit Tart, 157
    Fruit Freeze, 166
    Mixed Fruit Breakfast Smoothie, 122
    for skin hydration, 334
Full by Living Proof Root Lifting Spray,
    309
Fusion Beauty PrimeResults Anti-
    Redness Primer, 326

G

GABA, in relaxation drink, 277
Games, fusion, for calorie burning, 114
Garlic
    Honey-Glazed Pork with Garlic
        Mashed Potatoes and Roasted
        Broccoli, 74
    raw, benefits of, 241
Gastroesophageal reflux disease (GERD),
    252
Genetically modified organisms (GMOs),
    255–59
GERD, 252
Ginger lemonade, workout benefits from,
    103
Giorgio Armani Acqua Di Gioia perfume,
    349
Giovanni Colorflage Perfectly Platinum
    Color Defense Shampoo and
    Conditioner, 317
Glo Minerals Lid Primer, 328
GMOs, 255–59
Goodman, Myra, 286
Grains, whole, as Active Calorie food, 68, 69

Granola
    Breakfast Parfaits, 123
Graves' disease, 282
Green tea. *See* Tea, green
G-spot, 45
Guided imagery, during medical
    treatment, 24
Gum sensitivity, hormones and, 48

H

HAES, for breaking dieting cycle, 112–17
Hair
    aging and, 307
    flyaway or frizzy, products for, 310, 317
    gray
        almonds preventing, 332
        attitudes about, 312, 315
        cause of, 313–14
        celebrities with, 313, 315
        clothing and makeup colors with,
            314
        on eyebrows, 322
        products for, 316–17
        styling, 317
    improving health of, 300–301, 305,
        316
    quiz about, 296
    thinning
        causes of, 308–9
        products for, 309
        styling, 311–13
        treatments for, 310–11
Hair color. *See also* Hair, gray
    anti-aging, 299, 300
    foods boosting, 329, 334
    products for, 315, 316–17
    for thinning hair, 313
Hair conditioner, 316–17, 316, 335
Hair mask, yogurt as, 333
Hair removal. *See* Shaving

Intuitive eating, in Health At Every Size movement, 112, 115, 116
Iodine deficiency, 280
Iron
    for hair health, 300, 310
    sources of, for vegetarians, 243
Irritable bowel syndrome (IBS), 56–57
Itchy skin, treatments for, 335

J

Jackie Warner's Personal Training DVD, 193
Jergens Ultra Healing Extra Dry Skin Moisturizer, 335
Jin Shin acupressure, 54
John Frieda Full Repair Touch-Up FlyAway Tamer, 310
Joico Clinicure Lifting Foam Volumizer, 309
Joint pain, from aromatase inhibitors, 57–58
Journaling, for fostering contentment, 264–65
Julie's Organic Juliette Ice Cream Sandwiches, 251
Jump rope workout, 191–92
Jump squat, in week 4 strength circuit, 102, **102**
Just Label It Campaign, 258, 259, 259

K

Karma Organic Nail Polish Remover with Soybean Oil & Lavender, 343
Kava, in relaxation drink, 277
Kickback squat, in week 2 strength circuit, 96, **96**
Kickback squat with heel lift, in week 3 strength circuit, 99, **99**
Kickboxing cardio booster workout, 198–99

Kid foods, avoiding eating of, 83
Kidney damage, from colonoscopy prep pills, 21
Kneeling pushup, in week 1 strength circuit, 92, **92**
Krochet Kids International hats, 289

L

Labeling
    on egg cartons, 225
    of genetically modified foods, 258, 259, 259
Lactose intolerance, 219
Lancome Tresor in Love perfume, 349
Lasagna
    Tortilla "Lasagna," 153
Lashes. *See* Eyelashes
Lash-growth serums, 322
Laura Geller Blush-N-Brighten with Brush in Pink Grapefruit, 299
Laura Geller Waterproof Eye Spackle, 328
Laura Mercier Secret Camouflage, 298
Left ventricular assist device (LVAD), for heart failure patients, 3–9
Legs, improving appearance of, 189
Lemonade, ginger, workout benefits from, 103
Lemons
    Lemon Sponge Cake with Mixed Berries, 158
Lentils
    Curried Sweet Potato and Lentil Soup, 134
    Wild Mushroom-Lentil Burgers, 234
Level Naturals Shower Bomb, 335
Lidocaine gel, for reducing mammogram discomfort, 18
Linguine
    Shrimp Scampi Linguine, 73

Meatless Monday campaign, <u>240</u>

Meats. *See also* Beef; Bison; Pork

lean, as Active Calorie food, 68

Medical imaging tests

mammograms, 17–19

MRI, 23–25

radiation from, <u>20</u>, <u>280</u>

ultrasound, 19, <u>28</u>, 31–33

Meditation, 56–57, 265, 269

Melange Perfumes Solid Perfume
Blending Palettes, 349

Melanoma, 341

Melatonin, in relaxation drink, 276

Memory improvement, from
acupressure, 54

Menstrual cycle, hormones and, <u>48</u>

Mental acuity, hormones and, <u>48</u>

Meridia weight loss drug, dangers of, 106,
107

Metabolism boosters, 68, 72, 87

Migraines, acupuncture for, 58, 60, 62

Milk, fat-free, workout benefits from, <u>103</u>

Mindfulness meditation, health benefits
of, 56–57

MiniChill relaxation drink, 276–77

Minoxidil, for hair growth, 310–11

Modern Glass Water Bottle, <u>88</u>

Moisturizers

body, 305, 335

facial, 302–3

foot, 345

hand, <u>345</u>

when to apply, 301

Mondays

easing transition to, <u>271</u>

meatless, <u>240</u>

work hours completed on, <u>272</u>

Mood, scents improving, 348

Mountain climber, in total-body toner
workout, 197, **197**

Mouth drooping, concealing, <u>298</u>

MRI, 23–25

Muffin top, reducing, 205–6, **205–6**,
<u>208</u>

MultiDrink water bottle, <u>88</u>

Murad Acne & Wrinkle Reducer, <u>331</u>

Mushrooms

Baked Mushroom Risotto, 142

Vegetable Pancakes, 138

Wild Mushroom-Lentil Burgers, 234

Mustard

Grilled Rib-Eye Steak with Mustard
Sauce, 148

N

Nail polish

anti-aging effect of, 301

for pedicure, 345

speeding drying time for, 335

Nail salons, cleanliness of, <u>344</u>

Nasal spray, for nosebleeds, <u>24</u>

Nausea, acupuncture for, 58, 60–61

Neck cream, recommended, 304

Nelsons Pure & Clear Purifying
Cleansing Wipes, <u>331</u>

Neutrogena Tone Correcting Daily
Moisture SPF 30, <u>326</u>

Neutrogena Ultra Sheer Dry-Touch
Sunblock SPF 30, 340

New Balance 860 athletic shoe, <u>178</u>

Nighttime snacking, preventing, 81

Nitroglycerin, Viagra and, 40, 41

No-equipment total-body toner workout,
195–97, **195–97**

Non–GMO Project seal, <u>256</u>

Nosebleeds, nasal spray for, <u>24</u>

Not A Perfume, 350

Nuts

as Active Calorie food, 68

almonds, as beauty food, 334

Sustainable food, locating, <u>290</u>

Sweet potatoes

    Chicken–Sweet Potato Stir-Fry, 146

    Curried Sweet Potato and Lentil Soup, 134

    Sweet Potato Gratin with Pecan-Crumb Topping, 143

Swim, in Ballet Boot Camp Challenge, 186, **186**

Swissco Emery Glass Nail File, 344

Synthroid, for thyroid disease, 281, 283

T

Tarragon

    Warm Potato Salad with Tarragon, 129

Tart

    Fancy Fruit Tart, 157

Tartine

    White Bean "BLT" Tartine, 156

Tata Harper skin-care products, 291

Tea

    as beauty food, 329

    green

        in Active Calorie Diet, 68–69

        for relaxation, 276–77

        workout benefits from, <u>103</u>

Tea bag, for split lips, <u>24</u>

Teeth, yogurt protecting, 333

Testosterone, for sexual desire in men, 44

Thyroid cancer, <u>280</u>

Thyroid disease

    diagnosis of, 282–83, <u>283</u>

    hair loss from, 309

    patient stories about, 279–82

    prevalence of, 279

    protective measures against, <u>280</u>

    types of, 282

Thyroid-stimulating hormone (TSH), 281, 283

Thyroid supplements, avoiding, <u>280</u>

Toe lifts, for strengthening foot muscles, 175

Toenails, pedicure for, 343–45

Tomatoes

    Beans with Herbed Tomatoes and Goat Cheese, 141

    cooked, benefits of, <u>241</u>

    Tortilla "Lasagna," 153

    White Bean "BLT" Tartine, 156

Tortillas

    Tortilla "Lasagna," 153

Total-body toner workout, no-equipment, 195–97, **195–97**

TouchBack BrowMarker, 322

Transvaginal ultrasound (TVU), for ovarian cancer screening, <u>28</u>, 31–33

Treadmill fat burner workout, 194, <u>194</u>

Triceps kickback, in week 1 strength circuit, 93, **93**

Triceps lifts in crescent lunge, in Ballet Boot Camp Challenge, 185, **185**

Triple-duty bent-over row, in belly blaster workout, 216, **216**

Triple-duty butt kicker, in belly blaster workout, 215, **215**

Triple-duty cheerleader press, in belly blaster workout, 213, **213**

Triple-duty chest press, in belly blaster workout, 214, **214**

Triple-duty pullover and crunch, in belly blaster workout, 216, **216**

Triple-duty side leg-lift crunch, in belly blaster workout, 217, **217**

Triple-duty skater side twist, in belly blaster workout, 215, **215**

Triple-duty squat and curl, in belly blaster workout, 214, **214**

TSH, 281, 283

Turnips

    Roasted Vegetable Soup, 137

TVU, for ovarian cancer screening, <u>28</u>, 31–33
TV watching, limiting, on weekends, <u>268</u>
Tweezerman Brow Shaping Scissors & Brush, 323
Tweezerman Pedro Too Callus Stone, 344
Tweezers, first-aid uses for, <u>24</u>

U

Ultrasound
    for breast cancer screening, 19
    for ovarian cancer screening, <u>28</u>, 31–33
Umberto Beverly Hills Volume Shampoo, <u>309</u>
Under-arm flab, reducing, 207–9, **207–9**, <u>208</u>
Unwind relaxation drink, 276
Upper GI series, as alternative to endoscopy, 22

V

Valerian, as sleep aid, 277
Vanilla beans
    Chocolate Cherry Cupcakes with Vanilla Bean Frosting, 164
Vegans
    iodine deficiency in, <u>280</u>
    stories of, 241, 243–45
Vegetables. *See also specific vegetables*
    as Active Calorie food, 68, 69
    cooked vs. raw, benefits of, <u>241</u>
    Roasted Vegetable Soup, 137
    for skin hydration, 334
Vegetarianism
    benefits of, 240–45
    increase in, 239–40
Vegetarians
    protein and nutrient sources for, <u>243</u>
    recipes of, <u>245</u>
    types of, <u>242</u>

Veins, spider, on legs, 189
Ventilatory threshold, fat burning and, 86
Viagra, 39–41, 44–46, 107
Vichy CelluDestock, for cellulite, 189
Virtual Active DVD, <u>193</u>
Virtual colonoscopy, 21
Vitamin B$_{12}$ sources, for vegetarians, <u>243</u>
Vitamin C, for skin health, 333
Volunteering, on weekends, 269
Vomiting, acupuncture for, 60–61

W

Waffles
    Cocoa-Espresso Waffles, 125
Walker, Amanda, 288
Walking, finding opportunities for, <u>198</u>
Walnuts
    Chicken with Walnuts and Spinach, 147
Water
    in Active Calorie Diet, 69
    calorie burning from, <u>87</u>
    herb- and fruit-infused, <u>276</u>
    for skin hydration, 334–35
    for sunburn, <u>338</u>
    during workouts, <u>103</u>
Water bottles, recommended brands of, <u>88</u>
Water temperature, for beauty treatments, 335
Web surfing, limiting, on weekends, <u>268</u>
Weekends
    rules for enjoying, 267–69, <u>268</u>
    transitioning to work after, <u>271</u>
Weight gain, foods causing, <u>75</u>
Weight loss
    dieting for (*see* Dieting)
    eating tips for, <u>87</u>
    exercise for (*see* Exercise; Workouts)
Weight Loss Cookbook, 118–67. *See also specific courses and recipes*